The

Heroine's Journey

A Tale of Love, Forgiveness, and the Implications of Universal Laws

Gail Lynn

Dear Reader,

Everything happens for a reason! Find the reason and become the heroine (or hero) of your own life!

With love,

Gail Lynn

Back Cover Photography: A special thank you to Lance @ Living Moments Media, Maui, Hawaii for bringing out the heroine in the photoshoots. https://livingmomentsmedia.com

Editing: Niki Patino www.nikipatino.com

~

For my children. In my deepest, darkest hours, it was you that kept me going. Thank you for never turning your back on me. I love you forever.

Table of Contents

~Prologue~

The Heroine's Journey

After four years of suffering from Lyme disease, I made the decision to go full speed ahead with my healing journey to reach the finish line. It was May of 2017 when I made the plan. I was going to Hawaii for a summer healing journey, of alternative health measures that would complete my understanding of how to heal my body. My journey began on the island of Maui at the Hay House Writer's Workshop, and then I went on to seek the services of a shaman. After that, I went to the Big Island of Hawaii for further help on my healing journey. My intention was to complete the healing needed in my body through alternative health modalities, whatever that entailed. I stopped believing in Western medicine. My only goal was to find the missing piece of something, but even I did not know what that was.

I began with God. As a child, I was told that all things are possible with God. I remember sitting with my grandmother at her kitchen table as she read to me from her Bible. To this day, I still remember her pointing out one verse, in particular, Philippians 4:13, "I can do all things through Christ who strengthens me." It is worth repeating, but also understanding, for there are secret meanings in scripture.

I can do ALL things through Christ who gives me strength. It does not say that I can do SOME things. It says ALL things. And who, or what, is Christ? Remember that.

I urge you, Reader, after finishing this book, peruse my recommended reading list written by my mentors and if you are not already familiar with the work of these authors, go and find them. See who you are drawn to, and follow that gut intuition. Do your own research about how their work is related to Hinduism and Buddhism and other religions and cultures from around the world. See for yourself how their work connects to your life, to healing, to creating the life we desire. See how it connects to the Bible and other ancient texts from all around the world. Discover for yourself how these teachings relate to the divine field of energy that permeates all around us that some call God, Spirit, Source, or Divine Intelligence. There are many names for this All-Knowing Energy, and behind each name is the essence of LOVE. Love is what binds us all together, and it is this Source, this unified field, that keeps us connected even when we feel separated.

~

Although I never had the pleasure of meeting Wayne Dyer before he passed into the spirit world, he speaks to me often. And like the title of one of his books says, *I Can See Clearly Now*. Wayne was with me for the whole summer I spent in Hawaii. He brought a doctor into my life, one of his own doctors, while I was sitting on an airplane waiting to take off in Buffalo, New York to head to Maui. I needed a doctor, not for treatment, but to offer something else. Whether you say it was God or my angels or Wayne's doing, I was placed in a seat right next to a doctor who knew Wayne. Miracles do happen.

As you read my story, *The Heroine's Journey*, I invite you to consider where YOU are on your own journey and what chapter of life YOU are living right now. This journey is not just my story, but it is YOUR story as well. The finer details may be different, but it is the structure of life as we proceed from birth to death of this physical body. Moses, Jesus, Buddha, Krishna; all the great teachers from around the world came to understand life in this way and each culture around the world has individuals who know this, yet each has a different way of saying it.

The Heroine's Journey will demonstrate to you how we are all connected, all of us, all over the world, as One. It will prompt you to keep learning, keep discovering, keep healing, keep loving. It will remind you and give reason to why the greatest commandment is to love the Lord your God with all your might. As Jesus said, "The Kingdom of God is within." I began to consider the notion that he was really telling us that we need to love ourselves more, which is exactly what this journey allowed for me.

In this year of 2020, in this unprecedented time of a worldwide pandemic, now more than ever it is imperative that we all begin to see more clearly the revelations that are before us. It is more important than ever that we begin to love ourselves more and our neighbors more. It is important that we recognize and use our power to lift others in love and contribute to a better world. As more people come to understand that by blessing others, we too become more blessed, and only more good will come.

If you are ready and willing to seek the truth, the truth will set you free. YOU are more powerful than you know. Your divine birthright is that of peace, love, happiness. It is your birthright to have all that you need and then some!

Dear Reader, I wrote this book for you. I wrote this book because I learned the secret of healing the physical body of illness, of creating a beautiful life, of having wishes come true. It is my goal to help alleviate the suffering of humanity, to help those who feel lost or burdened or sick.

My story is living proof that we have the power to heal our own illnesses. We have the power to be, do, and have anything that we want in life. It is all in our hands. And as you begin to understand and apply the Universal Laws, the laws of nature which combine science and spirituality, you too will become the hero or heroine of your own life.

I finally understand that the struggles which I endured in life were to teach me lessons about loving myself and others unconditionally AND about forgiveness.

So dear Reader, as this story nudges you, tugs at your heart, makes you wonder, know too that it will put you on a quest to find your own answers that you may not even know you are looking for.

So, grab a pen and begin reading! Mark up the book with your thoughts and feelings as you go. Write down any synchronicities or "Aha!" moments you have. See your own life stages mapped out and visit the work of the author, Joseph Campbell for his version of the journey, *The Hero with a Thousand Faces*. As a spiritual teacher, Ram Dass once said, "We're all just *walking* each other home."

As you read, remember thoughts are things. What we think about, we bring about. Think on things positive and you will bring in more positive experiences. Think on things negative and you will bring in negative experiences.

In the body, great health is available to all, no matter what your genes or family history. Your body is a temple, treat it so. Your biology is in your belief.

Our soul, or spirit, is connected to the Divine Intelligence. When we connect deeper with this field of divinity, the unified field, the divine connects deeper within us, co-creating more loving, kind, generous experiences.

Life is full of good health, wealth, and happiness. Death is disease, error, misery, and pain. Our life is an outward expression of our thoughts, words, and deeds. How are you showing up to live every day? What do you believe about life?

4

As we ask, so shall we receive. Together with the field of potential, WE create our life.

WE are the CREATOR.

I love you,

~1~

An "Ordinary" Life

Some of us have grandiose stories while others not so much. It's all relative anyway. But no matter how tragic or simple they are, our stories are meant to be shared with others. Yes, MEANT to be shared. If we all kept our stories locked up inside, we would never learn from each other. We would never grow. Our stories lead us to bond with others, to foster an understanding of the world around us, and to open us to healing as we see others who have gone before us along a similar path. Stories inspire us and give us hope for better days ahead.

If you are anything like me, you may have spent many months or even years contemplating life, wondering when it all began, or perhaps even where you went wrong. You've probably also wondered about the pain you've experienced, the wounds in your heart, or thoughts that have made you feel less than worthy.

My own conclusion to these ponderings is that it all began before I was even born into this world. I believe that my cells have carried into this lifetime many of my parents' fears and self-defeating narratives that I sponged up while in the womb.

I believe that the fears and lack of self-worth that I've experienced my whole life began at conception when the sperm of my father united with the egg of my mother and begat the cells that bore me. Only recently have I heard their life stories, and had I known earlier, could life have been different? Knowing our parents' history is important. NOT their sickness or tendency for illness, but rather their life experiences and emotions. For what happened to our ancestors, both the good and the not so good, are in us.

I can look back at my life now and see how I carried a part of my mother's fears, insecurities, and pains into my own life, bearing these wounds year after year, not understanding what they were or where they came from. Then, I contributed to them with my own experiences as well. Learning about cellular memory prompted me to ask my father about his childhood experiences also. I never knew his story. I never knew he was a child hiding in caves with my grandmother during the war. I never knew he rode off on a donkey with a stranger, trekking across Sicily to go work as a servant on a farm to help buy food for the family at the young age of eight.

The foundation upon which I built my life contained feelings of fear, depression, anxiety, poverty, unworthiness, despair, and failure. I built my life upon these feelings and experiences that were ingrained into my DNA by my parents. Then as a young child, around the age of four, I began to add my own experiences to that foundation of misery. That is when The Fear Miser was birthed in me.

~

My dad is angry one evening and there is a lot of yelling between my mom and him. We, or my mother, did something wrong. I don't know exactly what it was, but it isn't long afterward that we move out and my dad is no longer a part of our lives (not for a long while anyway). We move in with my grandparents until Mom finds an apartment for us. My sister, at seven years old, is one of my caretakers. She is two years older than me. She also helps take care of our little brother who is three years younger than me. Yes, I am the middle child, for a while.

I remember starting kindergarten and crying a lot. I always want my sister next to me. I think with Dad no longer around, I am afraid the rest of my family was going to leave me, too. He moved three hours away and I spent a week with him in the summers.

The story that I tell myself for many years was, "If you do something wrong, make someone mad, they will leave you." This becomes a core wound and enabled both a search for love in all the wrong places as well as a fear of abandonment. I refer to this core wound herein simply as The Fear Miser. The Fear Miser is like the little devil that sits on your shoulder whispering words that you are not worthy and pointing out all the things in life to be afraid of, yet the innocent child within wants to love, needs to be loved, but doesn't know where to find it. The Fear Miser evolves with me over the years creating havoc in my life, pointing out all the bad in the world, telling me I'll never be good at anything, reminding me I come from poverty and would stay there.

~

The Fear Miser comes to me one night to remind me of my unworthiness. Mom hires a teenage boy to babysit us while she goes out. Shortly after she leaves, there is a knock on the door and three other teenage boys walk in. They play music and sit at a table in the kitchen with playing cards. Peering into the kitchen, I hear the "twish" as the red, white, and blue can opens.

The next thing I know, I'm told to get back to bed. Climbing up to the top bunk, one of them follows behind me. He begins to undress me as the others laugh. Sitting naked, I am scared and ashamed.

~

To this day, I have never spoken about that night with my mom or my siblings. I do not recall exactly how long we lived at that address, but it wasn't long because the house caught fire and burnt to the ground. The man in the downstairs apartment fell asleep with a cigarette in his mouth. We lost our home and all our belongings. Fear, loss, and abandonment followed me.

~

Mom finds a new house across town, but this time her boyfriend and his three kids move in with us, too. The neighborhood is filled with kids, but for some reason, I like to be alone. I walk up and down the block admiring all the houses. At one end of the street is a large brick house. It looks like a palace.

I often stroll by and observe the old man working in the gardens. One day as I stand watching him from the sidewalk, he asks if I want to help with the rose bushes. I kneel beside him and grasp a weed to pull. I yank so hard I almost fall over backward. Pieces of dirt fly everywhere, including my hair and mouth. Sputtering, I feel embarrassed. The old man chuckles and says something about going to get a cold drink.

"Follow me," he says.

Inside the house are dark wood cabinets. I feel like I'm in a castle. I'm in awe as I stare into the dining room where a table sits covered with lace. Chandeliers glisten in the sun that streams in through the windows. I have never seen such beautiful things. Walking into the kitchen, I notice the shiny, speckled counter and two beautiful glasses. The old man starts to pick up the glasses, but then instead places them down, turns around, and walks towards me.

Stopping in front of me, I notice a smell, like my grandpa after a day in the garden. Dirt has a smell. The closer he gets, the smell gets stronger, and I become more nervous. An unsettling feeling washes over me. I remember this feeling vividly every time The Fear Miser returns.

He reaches down and puts his arms around me as an awkward feeling shoots up my spine. His suspenders are cold and hard against my bare arms. I stand there stunned, not knowing what to do, wondering why he is hugging me. Suddenly, he leans down and kisses my lips. Although taught to respect my elders, I still don't think this is right. With my heart racing, I squirm out of his arms.

"I have to go," I say as I sprint out of the house. I run the whole way home, shove the front door open, and race straight up to my bedroom.

~

I don't remember if I cried or not. I don't recall what happened after that other than feeling confused and wondering what I did to bring that on. As I think about that day now, it makes me sad for that innocent little girl who, once again, thought she had done something wrong. I felt dirty and ashamed and wanted to hide. I was afraid to tell anyone for fear I would get in trouble.

~

Not more than a year or so later, we move back across town again. Mom starts cutting my hair shorter and I am often mistaken for one of the boys. I am becoming rough and tough. I play with snakes and footballs and mud. Perhaps I am afraid to be a girl.

One night while playing a game of kill the carrier with the neighborhood boys, it's dark and I mistake a pine tree for my stepbrother and try tackling the tree. I end up in

11

the hospital screaming while strapped to a board while the doctor stitches up my mouth.

After a few weeks of healing up, the boys decide to build a fort underneath an old, abandoned house in the neighborhood. I want to join them. Climbing through an opening of deteriorated bricks in the foundation of the house, we are overcome with darkness. Here is where we have our club. The ground is cold. It smells like dirt.

The boys I am with don't care that I'm a tomboy. First, we play a game of truth or dare. One of the boys has a dare, and before I know what is happening, I am forced to the ground, flat on my back. I squirm and roll side to side trying to get away from his grip, but I am not strong enough. The others help him and hold me down as my shorts are pulled down. The two older boys hold me down as the other one takes off his clothes. They use me to teach him how to have sex.

I am a pawn in their game.
Meaningless. Worthless.
Dirt.

~

I was never the same after that day in the cold, dark crawl space. My motto became, "Trust no one." I was only a child, like an old rag doll, to be used and abandoned.

~

Around this time, I begin developing nervous ticks. I start pulling on my eyelashes, and before I know it, every single one of them is plucked out. When everyone laughs at me, I go to look in a mirror and notice what I have done.

I am anxious and afraid every time we have a babysitter, and pulling on my eyelashes somehow soothes me. After my eyelashes are all plucked out, I move on to my eyebrows. Everyone laughs at me and asks what

12

happened. During an eye exam at school, I decide I will fake the exam so I can wear glasses to cover up my eyes. I go home and tell my mom that I can't see very well and that I need to have my eyes checked by a doctor. I fake my way through that exam as well and come home with a pair of gold-rimmed glasses that will hide my eyes, or rather, that will hide the shame that I feel.

After a while, my eyelashes and eyebrows grow back. I get smarter and begin pulling on my hair instead. Every time I am hurt, left with a babysitter, smell dirt, hear the "twish" sound of a beer can opening, I become anxious. Reaching up behind my right ear, I begin by circling my hair around my finger. Next, I rub my scalp and pull the long hair away from my head as I release the fear, the anger, the shame. It's not long before bald spots begin appearing on my head.

I look funny. I hate myself. I have no way to hide the bald spots on the back of my head. I feel so unloved, so ashamed. I feel alone. Eight-year-old me does not know how to tell my mom what I am feeling or why. She is a single mother of three, finding her own way. I do not want to give her more problems. I do not want to make her mad. I do not want her to leave me abandoned as my dad did. The Fear Miser controls my life. The need for love and affection battle against this dark force within me.

~

As time goes on, advances by both boys and men continue. We move to the country to share a house with my grandmother. Then puberty hits and I begin developing breasts. Not knowing any better, most of the summer I walk around my house in my bikini thinking nothing of being half-naked until Mom's boyfriend begins making inappropriate comments.

Folding laundry one night, he enters the living room with his breath reeking of alcohol. Angry that the laundry isn't already folded, he leans in closer forcing me to look at him. Then suddenly turning a smile on, he reaches out and grabs me with the same sort of forced embrace that I have felt numerous times before. Planting his lips on mine, he shoves his tongue into my mouth.

Fortunately for me, my grandmother is home in the back apartment. Hearing her voice as the backdoor opens is a godsend. A night of chaos ends as two police cars pull out of the driveway, Mom's boyfriend in tow. I am ushered away to a friend's house. I don't see Grandma again until the next day.

~

It was years later that Mom finally revealed he had pushed Grandma and she fell and sprained her wrist. It was then that she also revealed the truth about her black eye and other "mishaps" she had over the years with him.

~

Now in middle school, I begin dating, of course always the older boys. Each one wants to show me how much they "love" me. Led to a camper in the field next to his family home, one boyfriend explains how he learned about sex from his parents and would teach me. "Let me show you how much I love you," he says. Meanwhile, I keep wondering, *What is love?*

~

The physical and sexual abuse continued throughout my college years and young adult years. My first time away from home was when I went to Fort Lauderdale, Florida, for a semester of college. I was a down-home country girl going to college in a party city. The excitement was too much, and I went running back home into the arms of another high school boyfriend.

I wasn't even home for six months when I became pregnant with my first child. Although we decided to marry, love still escaped me. Angry and bitter about his own childhood upbringing, being a dad was the last thing on Joseph's mind. We fought about money and his hobbies and not being home for our family. His way of showing love was no different than all the others. After two children and two years of abuse, I decided to divorce him and become a single mom. I was now on my own trying to love the two beautiful boys that I had brought into the world.

I didn't know anything about being a mother. They didn't teach that in school, and I didn't have a role model to follow. I was still learning about love.

Having moved into housing for those with financial need, I tried to create a home for me and my boys. A year passed and I began dating again. Laughing over a video game at a local pub, Stan, my date, asked me to drive him home. He had too much to drink. Helping him up the stairs became a struggle. He began telling me how much he loved me, and we both laughed so hard I about dropped him as I said, "Yeah, I've heard this story before."

After much courting and flowers and Sunday drives with my boys, my relationship with Stan flourished. Next came a house we built together with the boys and then a wedding and then a new baby. I finally had something that resembled the kind of love that I was looking for. I told myself I would get it right this time. I told myself that this time I would not be abandoned. I would create the perfect home for Stan and our family.

We began taking our children to church every Sunday and afterward sharing meals and conversations about God with other young families. We created an annual tradition of joining other families each summer at church camp and surrounding our children with the teachings of God. I went on my first mission trip, meeting the people of Guatemala with service and love.

I did everything possible to create a "perfect" family and protect my family unit. I stayed home and started a daycare and contributed to the family even greater financially. After my daughter reached school age, I decided to go back to school myself and have a career. With all three of our children in school, I had more time to attend classes at the local University.

Every holiday I invited family, extended family, and friends to join us for dinner. I even invited people who had no other place to go. I was tending to everyone's needs. I wanted so much to fit in, to be liked, to have the perfect family. I wanted the "white picket fence" family. I kept giving what I thought was love. Whenever someone needed something, I gave. I was the supermom who did it all. I cleaned. I cooked. I cared for the children. I became a soccer mom and a coach and a Girl Scout Leader. I handled the bills. I entertained. I took care of the landscaping. I made everything pretty.

For ten years I gave to the point of exhaustion. I gave until I had nothing left to give. Then, the old feelings of not being loved began to creep in again. The Fear Miser returned. At first, I tried to hide the emptiness I was feeling. The Fear Miser reminded me that if I spoke up, I would be left abandoned. I simply stopped talking to my spouse. Stan and I started going days without talking to each other. Days turned into weeks and I began sleeping on the sofa.

For two years I survived like that until I finally broke down. "I don't feel loved," I told my husband.

We tried making it work, went to several counselors, but after a few more years of feeling unloved and alone, I found love in the arms of another man and asked for a divorce. The dreaded "D" word brought shame to me once again. Divorce was like a sickness, a symptom of someone feeling unloved. I needed to cure this sickness in me.

I vowed to myself to never try my hand at marriage again or ever trust anyone with love. Spending time with my children and attending their school and sporting events was my life.

~

As my own children began to get older, they didn't need or want Mom around as much, so my career became my life. By this time, my oldest son, James, was in college, my middle son, Josh, went to live with his dad, and my daughter, Sara, was home but spending more time secluded in her bedroom. The family that I loved more than life itself had fallen apart, and I did not know why or how.

I began to turn to my friends for more support. Having girlfriends to talk with and share highs and lows in life helped me get through some of the most difficult times I faced. Meanwhile, I was doing everything I could to shut out the pain of feeling unloved.

Then, one summer night while at a benefit, I was dancing with my girlfriends when I noticed a dark-haired man across the dance floor staring at me. I tried to look away, but each time I glanced over, he was still staring at me. He smiled and motioned for me to come over. I knew this game well, so I took my time and waited for the song to end before making my way to his side of the room. He looked me up and down and smiled.

"You know how to dance," he said with a grin. "I'm Bryce. What's your name?"

"Gail. Gail Lynn," I said, reaching out my hand.

We spent the remainder of the evening laughing and dancing together until it was time to leave. Walking me to my car, he asked, "Can I get your phone number? Would it be alright if I called you sometime?"

A few days later, I got the first call. He wanted to take me out for dinner. Each day thereafter he called, and we met for dinner, for a walk, or for a ride on his Harley.

A month had passed when he called and asked me about going to see fireworks on the Fourth of July. "It's like a little fair with vendors," he explained, "and they end the evening with fireworks. Do you want to go?"

That night was typical of a new relationship; conversations about things we liked or didn't like, and then as we began laying a blanket out to sit on for the fireworks to start, he stopped suddenly and stared into my eyes. Something was up. His big brown eyes were teary.

"What's wrong?" I asked.

But then the fireworks began, and we sat down. I looked over at him and again noticed his teary eyes. He reached for my hand and told me to watch the fireworks. Smiling, he looked up into the night sky. I leaned in and again asked.

"What's up, Bryce?"

"Nothing," he said. "It's just...well...I'm falling in love with you."

My heart skipped a beat. I sat there staring at him, not knowing if I had heard him correctly or if the sound of the fireworks had distorted his words. I must have looked as confused as I felt because he said it again.

"I love you."

That time I knew I heard him right, but I didn't know what to do or say, so I smiled.

"Thank you," I said.

I felt awkward. I wasn't expecting it. I wasn't prepared for this or ready to hear it. I had given up on love. I was just dating. I couldn't say it back to him. There was a voice inside my head that was telling me he was waiting for me to say it back, but I couldn't. I wanted to tell him what he wanted to hear, but I couldn't say it.

What is love? I thought. H*ow could he love me already?*

The night ended well, despite the jolt, but it put our relationship into a whole new arena that I wasn't ready for. Over the next few weeks, he began saying it more and more.

Each time we said goodbye, he said, "I love you" and I responded, "Thank you, Bryce." I didn't know what else to say. I didn't understand how he could love me.

He doesn't know me yet, I thought. *He doesn't know my past. He doesn't know my dreams or my hurts. I fail at loving people. You don't want me to love you. I don't know a thing about love.*

The first three months of our relationship were happy. We had so much in common. We took weekend getaways to wine country and went on excursions riding his Harley. Even though every weekend was spent living together at either his house or mine, in my mind we were just dating. I was always waiting for the other shoe to drop and for him to leave or stop loving me, just like all the others in my life had done. I was waiting for a sign from the Universe, from God, that HE, Bryce, was the ONE, that he could be trusted and would never abandon me.

That sign never came. What did come was The Fear Miser, abandonment, betrayal, and a breakup.

~

For three months we didn't talk, but then he showed up one day to mend the relationship. We were on another high of bliss for three months but then broke up again right after Christmas. It went like that. On again, off again. Our good times were filled with passionate love, dancing, and weekend getaways. But then something always arose that would result in disagreement and Bryce would pack up his bag and leave. Once, I came home, and his drawer in my bedroom was empty without even a goodbye.

We were crazy attracted to each other like bees to honey who needed its sweet nectar. Each time we got back together, I became even more addicted to that nectar of love between us. It was Valentine's Day in 2011 when he made a special dinner and then got down on one knee in his living room and proposed. I was so in love with him, yet at the same time, The Fear Miser whispered that he would abandon me again. Despite everything, I still said, "Yes!"

Bryce and I were ecstatic to be engaged. Some of our friends asked when we were going to tie the knot, but other friends questioned his commitment and warned me it wouldn't work.

"You really should take a year before setting any dates," said one friend. "He hasn't been able to commit to you for even six months, let alone be committed for a lifetime."

I had already considered the same thing. I shared my feelings with Bryce about waiting a year before setting a date. With our track record of breakups, I didn't want to go into a marriage predestined for failure. I wanted this to work, but I had hesitations about his level of commitment and ability to work through our disagreements.

We began talking about how we would join our lives and houses, but it soon became an area of conflict. I wanted us to live in my house since it was a place where I could easily continue having family dinners and holiday parties, but he wanted us to live in his house so he wouldn't have to drive 35 minutes to work each day.

My house seemed to be the most appropriate. My kids had never even been to Bryce's house, plus, all three of them were grown and living their own lives. James was a newlywed. Josh was fresh out of the US Air Force and bouncing between his dad's house, my house, and a friend's house. Sara was away at college and only home for holidays and breaks. Although they were grown adults now, spending time with my children and hosting family dinners once or twice a month was important to me. We had traditions that I wasn't ready to give up.

That year, like every year, I was hosting a family gathering at my home to celebrate the Fourth of July holiday. My favorite. Bryce and I had just returned from a weekend of camping that had not gone so well. All weekend, we were arguing about where to store the food in the truck to avoid attracting bears, and that turned into a fight. Many things became a fight with Bryce. He never met The Fear Miser, so he never really understood me.

He didn't want to dirty up the inside of his truck with a cooler, so he decided to put the food cooler in the back of the truck. Little did he know of my previous camping experience with a visit from a bear. Trying to explain, he brushed me off like I didn't matter. The Fear Miser turned into anger and then sadness as I questioned his feelings for me and why I would marry a man who disregarded my feelings.

On our way home from camping, I needed to stop at a store to pick up a few things for the picnic. "Hey, honey," I said. "Don't forget I need to stop at the store."

Still mad from our argument at the campsite, he continued on in silence.

"It's not like it's out of our way," I tried. "I don't know what the big deal is. I'll run in quickly and grab a few things, and you don't even need to get out of your truck." I hated how he made something so simple into a big ordeal. He pulled in and parked near the front entrance of the store.

"I'll wait here," he murmured.

I made a quick dash into the store to grab a few things and then rushed back out. He was texting someone on his phone as I hopped back into the truck.

"See," I said. "That took me, what, eight minutes? Who are you texting?" I asked him. He said nothing, but it left me wondering if he was hiding something.

Back at my house, I grabbed the grocery bags to bring inside as Bryce unloaded our camping gear. A few minutes later, he walked to the refrigerator and pulled out a beer. The "*twish*" made me stop in my tracks. I remembered that sound. A shiver went up my spine as I began prepping for a dish of antipasto.

Fill the pan with water, wash the veggies, get the cutting board. Like the hands ticking on the clock, I moved through the motions methodically. The day was already filled with strife, and I knew him drinking that beer would only make matters worse. Within minutes, he was in the refrigerator grabbing another beer. *Twish*.

He turned to me and asked, "Do you want any help?"

The first beer relaxed him a little, the first one always did.

"Sure," I said. "You can cut up the tomatoes while I finish washing the rest of the veggies."

By the time family and friends arrived, Bryce was on his fourth beer. He went from social butterfly to analytical observer within an hour, shifting between a happy talker to a silent observer. I could tell he was on the brink of starting a fight, so I paid no attention to him.

The day wore on. People came and went. I did my best to avoid any confrontation with him. I laughed with my kids and their friends and avoided Bryce. Eventually, things began to wind down and people were leaving to get ready for the fireworks. I considered just taking him back to his house and spending the evening with my kids and their friends, but I wasn't quick enough.

"Let's get the bike and ride over to the fireworks," he offered.

"I don't think that's a good idea," I said. "You've been drinking all day. Maybe I should just drive you home."

The mention of his drinking angered him.

"What the fuck do you mean?" he asked. "Drinking all day? I had a few beers. I'm fine. Let's go get the bike." He grabbed his keys off the counter and headed out the patio door. I followed behind him. Something didn't feel right.

"Let me take you home," I said. I reached for the keys, but he pulled away. The evening had settled in. I looked at Bryce then to the horizon. The voice in my head said, *No motorcycle!* My heart began to race. Feeling anxious, I sensed something bad was about to happen, so I reached for his keys again, but he yanked his hand away.

"You won't be taking me anywhere," he asserted. "I've had enough of this bullshit. I can just leave myself. You don't want to be with me? You want to hang out with those kids, then fine. Maybe I should take the ring back and let you go." He reached for my hand and started to pull the engagement ring off of my finger.

What is happening? I thought. *Has he lost his mind?*

"Is this ring even important to you?" he snarled. "Do you even want this?"

For a brief moment, he stopped and seemed to contemplate his next move. The ring was a symbol of our love.

I tried to yank my hand away, but he held on tighter.

"Don't do it, Bryce," I warned firmly. "You'll be sorry." I tried to pull back again, but it was too late. He pulled the ring off.

"You think you can dangle that ring in front of me like a carrot in front of a rabbit," I said, my steady tone edging up to a yell. "You think I'm going to jump just for a ring. You dare to take that off my finger and dangle it in front of my face? What is wrong with you? This is not love, Bryce! Keep your damn ring!" I grabbed my cell phone out of my pocket and called his sister to come get him.

"Your brother has been drinking all day," I told her, "and he's threatening to get on his Harley and go for a ride. Please come get him before he does something stupid."

"I'm on my way," she assured me. "Don't let him leave."

"You didn't need to go and do that," he spat. "I'm fine to drive. Just give me my keys."

"No, Bryce, I won't. Your sister is on her way. I promised I wouldn't let you leave."

He turned and walked outside and sat on the big boulder facing the road. Fifteen minutes later, a white suburban pulled in. I watched in slow motion as he hopped down off the rock and staggered to the vehicle. He opened the backdoor and slammed it shut. Through the window, I saw him put his head back on the seat as they drove off.

My heart raced. I ran inside and started pacing back and forth.

What just happened?

I looked down at my ringless finger.

How could he? I cried.

~2~

The Call To Adventure

My insides felt like a bubbling volcano about ready to erupt. I wanted to trust him, but just like I feared he would, he had abandoned me again. He abandoned *us*. I began sobbing as a stream of thoughts escaped in a garbled mess.

"Why?" I screamed. "Why does this keep happening to me?" There was no one there to hear me, no one to respond or answer the question that seemed to be the story of my life. "Why does everyone abandon me?"

My bursts of tears turned to outrage. I yelled at God, yelled at myself, yelled at the world. "WHAT'S THE USE OF THIS FUCKED UP LIFE? AM I SIMPLY A PAWN IN SOME SICK GAME?"

Nothing made sense. Tears flowed like rivers down my face as I sank to the floor.

"How could he make love so meaningless?" I whispered, losing myself in the darkness that had settled in.

Love was my addiction. I couldn't help it. I could think of nothing but it. I realized that my whole life I had been searching for someone to love me, ever since the moment my dad left.

When Bryce entered my life, I was protective of my heart. With two failed marriages, I was not interested in falling in love. I told myself I would never marry again. Ever. But over the course of the three years that we dated, I broke down. I accepted love into my life again, against all my fears. "Why didn't I listen," I scolded myself. I accepted an engagement ring when I wasn't even sure he would stay committed. I gave in and ignored my gut feeling.

My chest was heavy with the pressure of grief. Sobbing like a child, I walked out the patio door and looked up at the evening sky.

"Why?" I whispered. "Why does he give up so easily? Does he even know what love means?"

My heart pounded wildly against my chest. Walking to the edge of the deck, I grabbed hold of the railing. Dampness was settling in and a shiver went up my spine. My whole world was turned upside down. I looked up at the stars and wondered, *Why don't my wishes come true? Why can't I find love?*

I screamed at God again like a little child having a temper tantrum. "What did I do so wrong? Am I that unlovable?"

I was alone, again. Abandoned, again.

The sobs came harder as I fell to my knees. Somewhere inside me, a small voice whispered, *You are not lovable.* Pressing my forehead against the hardwood deck, I allowed the years of sadness to escape. My whole body shook as I cried.

The phone rang suddenly and interrupted the voices in my head. I stood and went to the patio door and looked inside at the clock. It was just after 8:00 pm. My first thought was Bryce. I hurried to the phone with a surge of panic feeling something was amiss.

Were they in an accident? Something happened, that voice said. Something wasn't right.

I looked down at the cell phone and read "James" on the screen. *Why is my son calling*, I wondered.

Holding my breath, I tried to answer, "H-ha, hello." I swallowed the lump in my throat and tried to speak it again, "Hello?"

"Hello, Gail," I heard Alycia, my daughter-in-law. "Are you all right?"

"No, I'm not," I admitted. "Bryce just left. We broke up."

"Oh, I'm sorry," she said. "I'm with James, but he's driving. Listen, I'm going to put him on speakerphone."

"Mom, are you alright?" James asked. "Did you hear the news?"

I couldn't quite hear him.

"I'm fine," I said. "You know me, always a fighter. I make it through. You heard already?"

I wondered how he knew that Bryce had broken off the engagement. "Bryce had too much alcohol to drink today," I continued. "He just walked out on me. He pulled the engagement ring off my finger and left. He wasn't able to drive, so I had to call his sister to come get him. How did you hear the news? This just happened." I began crying again.

"Mom," he said hesitantly. "Did you get a call about Josh?"

Every cell in my body froze. I tried to make sense of what he said, but more so, I heard the concern and the mention of Josh.

"What?" I asked. "What about Josh? Where's your sister? Is something wrong? Where's Josh?"

"Mom, I'm not going to tell you over the phone. I'll be right there. Are you alone?"

"Yes, I am. Why?"

Thoughts swirled in my head. My heart pounded. The Fear Miser rose like a monster from deep inside my stomach and set my body trembling. Something bad happened.

Sternly, I scolded my son. "James, you better tell me what's wrong. Tell me what happened! Do not keep anything from me, James. Tell me!"

I knew something was wrong with Josh. I could hear it in his voice. A mother just knows these things. Here I was worried about Bryce, and it was one of my own babies that I should have been worried about. I should have paid closer attention to the feeling in my gut.

"Damn it, James," I demanded. "What is going on?"

"Mom, I'm almost there. I'm just a few minutes away." I could hear the worry in his voice as he cleared his throat.

My heart felt so broken and defeated. I slumped down on the sofa crying knowing the night was becoming even more difficult. When the door finally opened, James walked in wide-eyed and serious. Running up to him, I searched his face for answers.

"What happened?" I asked fearfully.

Slowly, as if trying to make a point, he said, "Mom, we need to go. Get your purse and whatever else you need and get in the truck. We need to drive to the hospital. Josh had a motorcycle accident. They are flying him by helicopter to a hospital where they have a critical injury unit. We need to get there as soon as we can."

Gasping, I grabbed hold of his arm. "How bad?" I stammered. "How bad is he, James?"

"I don't know, Momma. Dad called. Said his helmet flew off. Said the emergency technicians wouldn't allow him to get close. He had a girl on the back of his motorcycle. We need to go."

I grabbed my purse, and we ran out the door.

Alycia was in the truck waiting for us. Placing her arm around me, she tried to assure me everything would be okay. "The police said his dad and stepmom are on the way. Do you want to call Sara and let her know?"

I fumbled around with my purse trying to fetch my phone. "Here, I'll dial it for you," Alycia said as she took the phone. James kept his eyes staring straight ahead. I could see the strain on his face and knew thoughts were scrambling through his mind as well. I tried to hold myself together as Alycia handed me the phone.

"Sara," I cried, my voice shaking. "Where are you? Who are you with?"

I got her friend on the phone and explained that her brother was in a terrible motorcycle accident and we needed her to meet us at the hospital.

"I do not want her driving," I explained. I tried to express how serious the situation was without alarming him or scaring Sara.

He put Sara back on the phone and I told her what I knew. I tried to keep calm so as not to cause any unnecessary fear, but every inch of my body was trembling. It was like no other feeling I'd ever had before. I was in shock and I just wanted to know that my baby was alive and was going to be okay.

My heart called out to my son, *Josh! Please be okay! God, please, take care of my baby!*

I hung up with Sara and called my mom next. I told her about the accident, that Josh was being flown to a trauma unit about an hour away, and I begged her to pray for him to be alright. Then I hung up before she could ask anything more.

I turned and looked at James. I could see the fear in his face. I turned to Alycia and asked her to get his father on the phone. "They are probably driving also," she said. "We'll be there shortly." She patted my leg trying to comfort me.

"He's going to be fine, Momma," James tried to reassure me.

I said nothing but instead silently prayed for God to be with Josh and the girl who was on the bike with him.

~

When we arrived at the hospital, a nurse led us to the trauma unit. As we got closer, I heard the sounds of a woman screaming. I froze. My heart plummeted wondering if the screams were coming from the girl who was on the bike with Josh. I heard the scream again. Yes, it was her.

I grabbed onto James' arm as we continued to walk through corridors. My stomach felt queasy and my head was spinning. Feeling faint, I looked up at James and held onto him tighter, afraid of what was coming. The screams from the woman got louder and louder. When we turned the corner, I saw Josh's father and a few others all pacing the hallway. The screams stopped, and then more sobbing began. I looked around anxiously hoping to judge the status of the situation by the look on everyone's face. I just wanted to know that Josh was alive and going to be okay.

Josh's dad was the first to come up to me and put his arms around me. It was the first time I'd embraced my ex-husband in many years.

"Hey," Joseph said. "Relax. He's alive and he's going to be fine. But you need to know what to expect when you see Josh lying on the gurney. You need to remain calm so he doesn't get upset."

Staring into his eyes, I stammered, trying to catch my breath between words. "Just…take me…to…my…son." Tears flowed down my face. My body shook as I held the sobs inside. Joseph took my hand and began to lead me to the curtain to where our son was being seen by doctors.

He stopped and looked down at me. "It's a bloody mess in there," he warned. "Are you sure you're ready for this? They haven't cleaned him up yet and the sight of him is pretty scary."

I simply repeated, "Let me see my son."

He reached up and pulled the curtain back. Fear pulsed through my body. I took a deep breath, wiped away the tears, and pushed past Joseph to see my son.

Stopping at the end of his bed, I gasped. "Oh, honey." The words trailed off as tears fell. I walked slowly up to his side with my eyes focused only on his face. I did not want to see what the rest of his body looked like. In my peripheral vision, I saw red, lots of red. That was not a good color in a hospital room, and there was so much of it.

"Oh, Josh," I murmured again. My heart grieved for my son lying there on the hospital gurney covered in blood. The room began spinning as I reached out to touch his hand.

Faintly, I heard someone demand a chair. The doctor came up to me and asked if I was okay. My eyes were blurry with tears, I turned back to look at my son. Reaching out and placing my hand on his, I didn't know what to say. No words came. I was just so happy to see his face, his eyes staring back at me.

"I'll be okay, Mom," he whispered. He tried smiling, but I could see through to the pain. I reached up and wiped a strand of hair off his forehead. Blood, sweat, and tears, *Josh has survived so much*, I thought. He made it through combat and several years of service. *Why now, God?*

Then another doctor entered and began speaking with Joseph and me about Josh's condition as if he weren't even there, as if he were an object that couldn't hear, like a car to be worked on. Trembling, I stood to meet the eyes of the doctor. Joseph reached out to help me up.

"I've got you," he said with concern on his face. For the first time, I looked at him with new respect. He was there, supporting me. We turned together and faced the doctor.

"We are waiting for the rest of the X-rays to determine the extent of damage to the fibula and the femur," the doctor stated. "The damage to the ankle is pretty severe and we will need to begin surgery as soon as we see what's going on. He continued describing the various bones and tendons that looked damaged, though his voice began to fade as I watched my son squirming in pain on the table. I brushed away Joseph's arm and went to Josh's side.

"Honey, what can I do for you?" I whispered, placing my hand on his. I tried to dismiss the sight of the blood-soaked blankets that covered him, but all I could see was red.

31

We spent the night sitting in the waiting room while Josh was operated on. It was the longest night of my life. By morning I felt drained, empty. My fiancé had broken off our engagement just hours ago, and now here I sat in the trauma unit while my son underwent surgery.

I began watching the second hand on the clock, counting each tick. At first, I prayed. Then, I tossed around angry words in my mind. Finally, my thoughts raced to Bryce and the events of the breakup and the pain that was in my heart. So many emotions played with me as I sat staring at people in the waiting room. People came. People left. And then, just as I looked to the entrance to see the newest arrival, there stood Bryce. He stared at me as if contemplating what to do next. Our eyes locked together, and he began walking towards me. I turned to look at Sara and the others who were seated around me. The look of disdain on their faces said it all. He wasn't welcome here. He hurt me; he hurt my family.

I stood and went to meet him before he could get any further into the waiting room where my family sat. With a cold empty stare, I asked him why he was there.

"I heard Josh was in an accident. I wanted to come and see if you needed anything." I could hear the sympathy in his voice, but it was too late. He broke off the engagement.

"No," I said coldly. "I need nothing from you. I need my son to be okay. And you can't help with that."

"Can I get you lunch?" he persisted.

"No, Bryce. Why do you care now? Last night you yanked the engagement ring off my finger. We are no longer a couple. You broke it off, remember? You've hurt me enough."

With tears in my eyes, I turned and walked away.

I sat back down next to Sara and laid my head on her shoulder. Closing my eyes, I thought about the events that had unfolded with Bryce the day before.

Bryce wanted to ride his Harley. If I had gone with him, I wouldn't have been home to receive the call. If I would have gone, maybe WE would have had the accident instead and that would have saved my son. Could I have prevented Josh's accident? Where did I go wrong, God?

I sat with my thoughts until it struck me that just as Bryce and I were arguing last night, I had stood at the patio door and looked out over the horizon to the little town of Bemus Point where Josh and his date were. Thoughts began reeling.

What if the tension that arose between Bryce and I was the result of my higher consciousness knowing that my son was going to get hurt? Or had it already happened? What if my motherly instincts knew that Josh was going to be in an accident before it happened? What if Josh had called out to me in the midst of his accident?

I couldn't handle or process my own thoughts.

Sighing, I reached over and took hold of Sara's hand. She looked down at me and with a faint smile gave me strength as she whispered, "I love you."

~3~

Resistance

After the surgery, the doctor came out and spoke with us to tell us that everything had gone well. Josh had a steel rod placed in his left leg from his hip to his knee and another placed from knee to ankle where a contraption of bars would protrude for several months until a future surgery would have it removed. It was all a blur.

After filling us in, the doctor finally took a deep breath and said, "Now would be a good time to go home and shower and get some rest. He will be in recovery for some time, and he'll be monitored for a concussion for the next 48 hours. If all goes well, he should be able to go into a regular hospital room in a day or two."

~

When we finally arrived home, I offered to grill some steaks and vegetables before the kids all went home. James went out to start the grill and then came back inside to where we were seated.

"Um, Mom," he said, "where's the grill?"

"What do you mean? You can't find it?" I said, laughing. "It's right where it always is, on the deck."

Walking out onto the deck, I looked around and saw that, sure enough, the grill was gone. I walked into the garage, around the side of the house, and to the front. It was nowhere to be found.

"That's odd," I said shaking my head in defeat. "It was here for our barbeque yesterday. Or was that the day before? You mean to tell me someone came here to the house while we were at the hospital yesterday and stole the grill? How can someone stoop so low? Like we need one more thing to go wrong in this family."

"I'm sorry, Momma. We'll just go home. I'm tired and just want to sleep anyways," James mumbled.

Alycia came over and put her arms around me. "Don't worry about it, Gail. You have enough on your plate right now. Whoever did that, they'll face their karma. We will check in with you in the morning to see when you want to go back to the hospital."

We said our goodbyes and they left. I turned to Sara and asked her if she was hungry.

"No, Mom, I'm good. Why don't you get some sleep? I'm tired, too."

Exhausted, I dragged myself over to the sofa and sat down. "Come sit with me for a few minutes."

Sara came and sat next to me. Resting her hand on mine, I stared at our hands, mesmerized, as the events of the past 48 hours rolled through my thoughts. I leaned my head against her shoulder and within minutes, I was falling asleep. Sara carefully stood, retrieved a blanket, and covered me.

The next morning, I awoke early, eager to get back to the hospital. I was sitting at the dining room table with my coffee in hand, staring out the patio door. The events of the previous day flooded my mind: July 4th barbeque, swimming, arguing with Bryce, and something about a motorcycle. My thoughts were interrupted by the sound of the phone.

"Hi, Alycia, you guys heading down soon?"

"Yes," she said. "We're just about ready to leave. Did you eat breakfast? James wants to stop for some food on the way to the hospital."

I looked at the clock. "As long as we're there by 8:00 am. I don't want to miss the doctor. Sara's still sleeping, so she'll need something to eat too. Just hurry." I was about ready to hang up when I heard Alycia continue.

"By the way, James got a text from one of his buddies. It was Bryce who took the grill. The guys were driving home from golf when they passed by the house and saw Bryce struggling to get the grill in his truck."

I sat in silence staring at the wall. The emptiness was all I felt.

Closing my eyes, I tried picturing Bryce coming to the house and taking the grill. I couldn't believe he would do that. That meant he left the hospital, where I sat waiting for my son to get out of surgery, to come to my house and take the grill that *we* bought together. Would he really do that? Now he had two at his house. I just couldn't believe it.

"I don't think he would do that, Alycia," I said. "It couldn't have been."

"Sorry, Gail. I didn't want to tell you, but you needed to know. James and I can help you get a new grill," she said. "Forget Bryce."

We hung up, and I went to look out the patio door to the deck. Something stirred within me. A picture flashed through my head of the evening argument with Bryce. We were standing here near the door arguing while my son crashed his motorcycle just over the hill. The image quickly dissipated as I heard Sara's bedroom door open.

Still looking sleepy, she walked into the kitchen. "Good morning, princess," I said as I went over and hugged her. "James and Alycia are on their way down. We're going to stop and get some breakfast on the way to the hospital. Can you get dressed quickly?"

"Yeah," she said, looking at me with concern. "How'd you sleep? You okay?"

"I'll be fine. I just want to get down to see Josh. Please get dressed so we can leave."

Everything was a blur. Grief took hold of me, yet I had to be strong for my son. The man who I thought was my soul mate had turned my life upside down. What was worse, was that my son had *his* life turned upside down as well. I had to pull myself together somehow and forget Bryce. Life was asking a lot of me.

My thoughts went back to the time when Josh was serving the US Military in Afghanistan. That was the last time I thought I had lost my son. We were on a skype session when sirens were blaring in the background, and the men in uniform scrambled out of their chairs and knocked them over right before the screen went black. There have been so many times that I have feared losing him. So many. I wondered how many more times God was going to taunt and test me. It felt as if an elephant was sitting on my chest.

I whispered to God, I pleaded, "Help me. I don't know how to handle this."

~

After days of traveling back and forth to the hospital and praying through surgeries, Josh was finally able to come home. It would be weeks before he could walk and months before he would have any sense of normalcy. We were warned that the transition would be hard, but there was much to be grateful for. I stepped into the role of changing bandages, administering medications, emptying bedpans, and talking with nurses and therapists. I was no longer just Mom but a nurse as well. For me, it was a learning curve between loving and letting go. I wanted so desperately to take away all of my son's pain, all of his fear and doubts. I wanted to take away the despair that encapsulated my home. I wanted to go back to the days when he was a little boy and wrap him in my love. I wanted to watch him laugh and play and see the world as kind and supportive. But instead, I had to pretend that I believed that all would be well, even though I wasn't quite sure if that was true.

As much as I tried to learn how to change the bandages, I could not stomach the sight of my son's bones sticking out of his body in awkward positions. I could not stand to see these foreign objects, steel rods and pins, protruding from his legs. Fear oozed out of me, and I'm sure my son sensed it. We were both grief-stricken. The home healthcare aides tried to give me lessons in nursing, but again, I felt like a complete failure. The words looped through my head over and over again, *You are a failure at everything.*

Josh wanted the bedroom blinds to stay closed. The dark bedroom was depressing, and like a damp basement that bred toxic mold, the energy in our home was toxic also. Day after day, Josh would lay in bed, unable to move, not wanting to participate in any conversation. I cooked breakfast, cleaned up the kitchen, cooked lunch, cleaned it up, did laundry, changed pads on bed, changed sheets, emptied bedpans, reminded Josh to take his meds, and repeated the same pattern day in and day out. I felt alone trying to fight off a monstrous dragon suffocating us both. I had thought I lost my son in a motorcycle accident, but next, I began to worry about losing him to depression. And me, I was ready to give up, too. I didn't know where to begin to put our lives back together. This failure as a mother was more than I could handle. I wanted it all to end. I wanted to leave my body. So began the thoughts of ways to end my life.

I found a bottle of vodka and walked outside to the patio. I slumped down on the step, unscrewed the cap, and put it to my lips for the first swig. I contemplated how to escape. Staring out across the valley, I began to consider how to end it. Then an idea popped into my head.

I'll walk to the top of my driveway, and just as a semi tractor-trailer comes barreling down the highway, I'll start crossing the road to my mailbox and fall in the middle of its path. It won't be able to stop in time.

I chugged the vodka until it was a third of the way down, then decided to go. As I stood, my stomach began swirling along with the trees in my line of vision. Tears slipped from the corners of my eyes.

I won't be missed. It'll be okay.

I walked to the edge of the deck, looking out at the massive backyard that was once filled with so much love and laughter. So many beautiful memories were made in that yard, yet it contained so much pain as well. I longed for those days when I was a simple mom, planning birthday parties and reading bedtime stories and rocking my babies to sleep.

I was jolted out of the memory by the sound of my daughter's voice.

"What are you doing, Mom?" Sara stood in front of me, face to face, with her hands on her hips. I stood there looking at her, surprised.

"I thought you had classes all weekend. When did you get home?" I felt suddenly ashamed. I melted like a baby with tears flowing down my cheeks as I babbled.

"I'm sorry, honey," I said, still holding the bottle of vodka. "I suck at being a mom. I can't even take care of my own son."

She looked from my face to my hand and then reached down, took the bottle away, set it on the deck, and hugged me tightly. Quiet sobs shook my body as she held me in her arms.

At that moment, she became the mother, and I became her daughter.

"I love you, Mom," she whispered. "Don't say things like that. You're doing fine. This is a lot to handle. Let's go inside and see what Josh is doing."

She led me inside to where my son was on his bed sprawled out on his back with his leg raised on several pillows. I climbed up on the bed beside him and pretended to watch TV. No words were exchanged. Sara climbed up on the bed and joined us. My heart felt heavy with despair and shame.

~

Hours later, my friend Jen called to see how we all were holding up. It had been a month since the accident, and I hadn't been out of the house or away from home since.

"You need to get out of the house," Jen said. "You need a break and some fun. Come join the girls and me for a fun night out."

"I'm not interested in a girls' night. What have you been up to?" I asked.

"Oh, come on. We're going to Lily Dale for Monday Night Circles," Jen persisted. "Maybe the medium will give you good news about your future life or maybe even a new man." She laughed. I knew she meant well, but I wasn't interested in meeting anyone.

"What's Lily Dale?" I asked.

"It's a spiritual community of mediums and psychics over on Cassadaga Lake. We go there for Monday Night Circles. They hold these events in their auditorium. They set up chairs in a circle for four or five people, and then one of the mediums comes to sit with us and gives each person a little reading," Jen explained.

"I don't know, Jen. I need to be here for my son. I don't know if I can get away."

Sara overheard me talking on the phone and interjected. She told me she would stay with Josh and I should go have fun with my friends.

"You can't just stay home and become a hermit," Sara chuckled. "You need a life. Besides, I'll be here. Josh and I can watch a movie."

I caved in and told Jen I'd join them.

"Meet us at 4:30 pm. I'll send you directions," Jen said. "We will walk down to Lily Dale once everyone gets there. Bring a lawn chair and snacks because we will have to sit in the long line for at least an hour before we get in."

I knew nothing about Lily Dale or their circles, but it didn't matter. I just needed out. I just wanted to forget everything for a while. Caring for my son allowed me to bury my own pain of the breakup with Bryce. It allowed me to bury my fears, bury my traumas, and to divert my attention once again so I didn't have to face the demons within. But in the quiet moments, I still wondered who I was and why I was here, why there was so much pain and fear in me. Questions like these taunted me.

Unlike the call that came to inform me of Josh's accident, the call from Jen was actually a godsend. Yes, I resisted healing the trauma from my past by focusing on my son, but the Universe kept pushing me onward into greater understanding. I wanted to stay home, but I knew I had to do something, not only for my sake but for my son's as well. It was time.

Sitting and waiting in line for Monday Night Circles, I contemplated what life would give me next. Little did I know, I was being pulled in through another door to a supernatural community of psychics, mediums, and healers.

~4~

Lily Dale, Mentors, and Mysticism

I knew when I was sitting there with my friends that the medium would pick me last to get a message. I was always good at guessing things like that, at *knowing* things and perceiving how people felt. I was always sensitive to people's thoughts and feelings.

When it was finally my turn to get a reading, he looked right at me without hesitation. "Why do you let that asshole get you all worked up?" he demanded to know. "You're too good for him."

The girls all broke out in laughter. I just sat there staring at this stranger, the medium. *How did he know that*? I wondered.

His name was Jim Barnum. "You're an empath," he told me. "When you learn to stop taking on other people's shit, you'll start getting along better." All the girls laughed again. This time, even I chuckled.

Hmmph, makes sense, I thought, but it was not what I expected from a medium. In a way that eased my tension, he continued speaking with me about the predicament my son was in and how both he and my ex-fiancé needed to grow up.

"Your son has been talking to a judge about a speeding ticket," he said to my surprise. "It wasn't his fault, but he needs to pay more attention to the roads. He'll have to pay a fine."

I sat there, amazed. *How does the medium know this stuff?* I wondered. *How does he know so much about my son and ex-fiancé?*

I nodded along in agreement to much of what he said about my relationship with Bryce and the weight I had been carrying for so long. He even hinted at knowing my secrets about wanting to end it all, though he was careful not to mention it outright, which I appreciated.

By then, the girls were on the edge of their seats listening attentively. I could tell they were just as surprised as I was.

By the time I left the Lily Dale auditorium, the hundred-pound rucksack that I had been carrying around for so long had disappeared. I hugged each of my friends. "Thank you for inviting me here tonight," I said. "It was a big help."

They all laughed and chimed in.

"We told you it would be good."

"You needed a night with the girls."

"And a medium!"

Now I had new things to figure out. I started by searching the word "empath" online when I got home that evening. As it turned out, I learned that an empath was a person with the paranormal ability to apprehend the mental or emotional state of another individual. Yes, that's me.

Another search led me to find Dr. Judith Orloff. She wrote, "Empaths are extremely sensitive, finely tuned instruments when it comes to emotions. They feel everything, sometimes to an extreme, and are less apt to intellectualize feelings. Intuition is the filter through which they experience the world. Empaths are naturally giving, spiritually attuned, and good listeners."

A door into the spiritual world had opened.

~

The next day I awoke and felt compelled to return to Lily Dale. I had never been one to go anywhere alone, so I reached out to several friends to join me, but no one was available. I had to make the choice to go it alone or stay home and resist this strange urge to return.

I mustered up the courage and made the drive to Lily Dale and learned more about this strange little community that was only fifteen minutes from my house. I wondered how it was that I had grown up in the area, spent most of my life there, raised my kids there, yet never knew about this special little place in the world.

As I entered the gates, I asked for advice on where to start. I was given their program of events and a map that would direct me to different places in the community. The attendant told me to park by the hotel and walk up the hill to begin my day at The Healing Temple.

"That seems to be the favorite place everyone goes to first. From there, just follow the crowd. Most of them will head to Inspiration Stump at 1:00 pm for messages from the mediums."

I did what I was told. As I walked up the hill, I began to notice a long line of people waiting to get into a little white church. There must have been at least a hundred people standing in the street waiting to get in. As I got closer, I saw a sign for The Healing Temple. I noticed people tying ribbons onto a tree in the front yard. Ribbons of all colors adorned the tree. It was beautiful.

I joined the line and began to eavesdrop on the conversations going on around me. One woman said she came here every summer just to attend the healing services. Another woman spoke about her friend with cancer that she was going to "sit for" today. The bald man behind me just stood there quietly, like me, taking it all in. I wondered what healing he needed.

As I got to the entrance, I let out a heavy sigh and released the tension that had crept up into my shoulders.

Making my way to a chair in the back, I felt a sense of peace like a warm blanket wrapped around me by the comforting arms of my grandmother.

Sitting quietly, I observed the others who came in. When it was their turn, the people walked to the front and sat at a bench where the healers in white jackets stood. Those in need of healing sat on the benches, and the healers went and stood behind them, closed their eyes, and put their hands on the shoulders of the person seated in front of them. When my turn came, I followed suit.

As I approached a bench, the healer smiled and motioned for me to sit.

"Are you seeking healing for yourself or someone else?" she whispered.

My whole life needed her prayers and healing.

"Both," I affirmed.

She whispered a prayer into my ear, then told me to close my eyes and relax. She put her hands on my shoulders for a minute or two then moved them to rest along the sides of my head. Heat emanated from her hands. They moved to my arms for a moment before moving down to my knees. In my mind, golden streams of light washed over me, as if she was purifying me of any filth. I silently thanked her repeatedly.

I'm not sure if it was the love that caused it or the gratitude, but a tear formed in the corner of my eye. I wanted to brush it away before it slipped down my face, but it was too late. Then another came and another. Feeling grateful for this woman, my heart opened to her. I opened my eyes to see her just as she reached for my hands.

"Thank you for letting Spirit use me," she said as she leaned in and whispered to me. "Have faith that whatever you need is on its way." She let go of my hands to signal she was finished.

Walking back to my seat, I decided to stay until the service was over. I closed my eyes and continued praying to

God. I thought maybe since this healer had prayed with me that this time my prayers would be answered.

Over the course of the next 10 days, I made time each day to steal away from home for an hour or two to go sit for spiritual healing. After the service, I walked up and down the streets and looked at the old houses. I went to Inspiration Stump and listened to mediums give messages to people in the audience. On several occasions, I sat at the quaint little coffee shop, Cup O' Joe, and observed the happenings of all the different people coming and going. This continued for a few weeks until summer ended, and the Lily Dale season was over. The gates into the community came down and the town became quiet.

It felt like another loss to not have this community to run to each day. I wanted more. Josh was making progress, my daughter was back in college, and I had gone back to work teaching fourth graders. Still, something was missing in my life. I found information about a development circle that was held on Tuesday nights at another spiritualist church that was just outside the gates of Lily Dale and decided to go.

I showed up one Tuesday night and bravely walked in. Jim Barnum was there, the same medium who I met at my first Monday Night Circle. He was hesitant to let me join.

"Do you happen to know anything about meditation or spiritualism?" he asked.

I stood and gazed at him, waiting for an answer to come to me, hoping he would simply welcome me to join in. I made some lame attempts to satisfy his questions until he gave in a little and began to explain the purpose of meditation. I listened for a minute until my eyes wandered over to a table of books beside me. I scanned the titles for something that would give me some insight as to what to do next.

He informed me there was a beginner's class I should consider, but then he gave in. "Go ahead and find a seat. We'll talk more after the class."

I looked over at the table of books again as I walked by. Dozens of books were meticulously organized by category. Healing, Mediumship, Crystals, Yoga, and so much more. I wasn't familiar with any of the authors, but I took note of various words to look up when I got home. Bhagavad Gita, Lao Tzu, Chakras, and Quantum Physics. I felt like I had stepped into a whole new world, and I felt stupid for not knowing what any of it was. I considered myself a pretty intelligent woman. I had a master's degree in Elementary Education and a certificate in School Building Leadership. This was beyond me though.

~

That winter began my initiation and crossing into the spiritual world. For the next ten months, I attended weekly classes with Lily Dale mediums, Jim Barnum and Shirley Calkins Smith. I was like a little kid in kindergarten learning all new subject matter. I listened to spiritual teachings that opened me up to new ways of thinking. New ideas began to emerge. Maybe I was a healer. Maybe I was a medium. Maybe I would finally learn what love was.

At Christmas, my brother, Darren, gave me my first spiritual book. It was by Eckhart Tolle, *A New Earth: Awakening to Your Life's Purpose*. Quickly absorbing its message, I read another book by Tolle, *The Power of Now*. Then I discovered Neale Donald Walsch and his work, *Conversations with God*. Various new age authors became mentors as I dove into reading about mediumship and healing. The world of metaphysics opened up to me one book at a time.

I dove into learning about meditation, mediumship, and Spiritualism. I learned about science and spirituality and the difference between being religious and being spiritual. Spring rolled around, and I began taking classes on spiritual healing.

When summer finally arrived and Lily Dale season of 2012 began, I was volunteering as a workshop coordinator to help the authors and presenters who came to teach. Every time I volunteered, my understanding of the spiritual world grew by leaps and bounds. I was being schooled on Reiki, chakras, crystals, pendulums, sacred geometry, reincarnation, and so much more.

Each class fit together like puzzle pieces as my eyes opened to a whole new world. One day, I overheard someone talking about the law of attraction and suddenly remembered reading a book about it by Rhonda Byrne, *The Secret*. At the time, it did nothing for me. I had never understood what the secret was in the book. I thought it was simply about getting what we wanted, like having a wish come true. But now, listening to these strangers talk about the law of attraction, I could make new connections between this universal law, metaphysical teachings, and biblical scriptures. I sought more answers.

~

Lily Dale gave me what I needed; a place to call home and a community of people where I felt like I belonged and was safe to learn from these mentors about this new world that I never knew existed.

As a public-school teacher with summers off, I volunteered to help with the Lily Dale program. I coordinated daily classes and became a spiritual healer at The Healing Temple. Despite my broken heart that I had buried, life was moving along again. My children were all busy with their own lives, and I was on my own journey of discovery.

In February, I was invited to speak at The Church of the Living Spirit. Excited and terrified, I prayed for guidance on what to say. It was a cold morning when I typed up words of inspiration to speak that coming Sunday. Streams of words flowed through my thoughts as I typed. I wrote and thought about the word "love" and the words "lack of self-worth" followed. Then came a vision of my mother.

I heard in my mind, *Like you, she didn't feel worthy.*

Questioning what that meant, I had a conversation with God in my head.

Why didn't she feel worthy? What does that have to do with me?"

A voice in me responded, *Her cells are in you.*

Then I saw a vision of my dad in an old black and white photo followed by the words "fear, shame, anger." What an epiphany that moment was as I heard those words. I immediately called my mom.

"Hey, sunshine," she answered. "You're calling awfully early. What are you up to this morning?"

I proceeded to tell her about my thoughts and the conversation I was having with God as I typed up my speech for church.

"Your grandmother was a stickler for a clean house," she confirmed. "Every time she came to visit, she would run her fingers over the furniture and comment about the dust. I never felt good enough for your father."

"Wow. That's interesting that God, or my thoughts, came up with that. Tell me about your relationship with Dad while you were pregnant with me," I said

After a good amount of time listening to her, I told her I had to get back to preparing my talk for church.

"What's your topic?" she asked.

"Love, of course. It's February!" We laughed and said goodbye quickly.

I sat there and suddenly realized my own struggle with worth was also my parents' struggle. I wrote my revelation into my speech:

> The Bible says, "The sins of the forefathers go three and four generations." I believe that is true. My mother's and father's mistakes, their so-called sins, or missing the

mark, are in me and my siblings. We have
struggled with self-worth our whole lives
like I'm sure many of you have at one point
in your life.

My talk that Sunday at church was very personal and
emotional. It hit at the core of not only my family but for
many others. Looking out into the audience, I could see it in
their eyes. Love for self was missing. What the world needed
and what hurting people all over the world needed was
unconditional love.

My own inner child, that little girl within, was still
battling with love for herself, yet here I was talking to an
audience about loving oneself. "THAT is the greatest gift we
have to offer others, and the greatest lesson we are learning,"
I concluded my talk that day.

~

Throughout the winter and into spring, I attended
services each Wednesday evening at The Healing Temple. I
was finding my way, becoming stronger emotionally, and
meeting more like-minded and caring people. I even began
sending good thoughts and love to Bryce each time I went to
The Healing Temple or worked as a healer in our Sunday
church services.

It had been some time since our paths crossed, but
then seemingly out of nowhere, Bryce showed up on my
doorstep. My heart softened when I saw him. When he
looked at me and smiled, I immediately forgave him for all
the hurt he had caused me and my family. I had endured the
most difficult time of my life on my own without him, yet
here he was showing up in my life.

We sat and talked for hours. When he left that night,
it was as if nothing had ever happened. We kissed goodbye
and made plans for dinner the next evening. Days turned into
weeks and we were a couple once again.

It was April when Bryce arranged for a weekend getaway to one of our favorite spots on Seneca Lake in the Finger Lakes. He had a knack for making things special when he wanted to, and this happened to be one of those times.

When we got to our hotel room, he rifled through his overnight bag. He turned to me with a big smile on his face as he took out a beautifully wrapped gift box.

"What's this?" I asked. It wasn't my birthday or any special occasion that would warrant a gift. Like a little kid with a present, I shook it and listened for something to rattle. Feeling giddy, I tore at the shimmering paper. I was excited to see what was inside.

"Oh, Bryce!" I exclaimed. "This is gorgeous!" I held the exquisite ivory lace dress against my body. "What's the occasion?"

"I just thought you needed a new dress for dinner tonight. I like seeing you in dresses," he chuckled. He had great taste in gifts as well as a talent for planning romantic evenings, though typically, the gifts and getaways were conditional. None of that mattered at the moment, though, he was happy and so was I.

Setting the dress down on the bed, I went and stood before him and took his hands. "Bryce," I whispered. I love you. I don't need gifts. I just need you. I'm so happy you're in my life again. We are meant to be together. Let's do it this time. Let's get it right."

Seeing the tears form in his eyes, I leaned in and kissed him long and hard. The same passion erupted as it usually did whenever we kissed. Our love caught fire. It wasn't long before we were side by side, naked and fully exposed to the afternoon sunlight coming through the window.

"Can we just capture this moment in a bottle?" I sighed.

"I love you," he said as he reached over and brushed the strands of sweaty hair off my face. "We're going to have a great dinner tonight and then more wine tasting tomorrow.

Let's shower and get ready. I want to see you in that dress."
He blew a few sweaty bubbles on my stomach before he
rolled off the bed with a smile.

~

We walked hand in hand into the Blue Pointe Grille
restaurant in Watkins Glenn. Bryce suggested that we grab a
cocktail and sit for a bit.

"I'd love a pomegranate martini before dinner."

"Why don't you grab that table over there," he
pointed across the room. "I'll get us drinks."

I went over and sat down. Watching him talk with the
bartender, he looked as though he was up to something. They
both turned and looked at me at the same time, then looked at
each other and laughed. My curiosity was piqued.

"What were you two talking about?" I asked when he
returned to the table. "I saw you guys looking at me."

"I told him to look at my sexy fiancée in her new
dress," he said with a sparkle in his eye.

"Thanks, honey," I blushed. "It's the dress. It's
gorgeous and I love it. But ... wait... what did you say?"

"I think you look even better with this on." He drew
my hand up and slowly placed our beautiful engagement ring
back on my finger.

Stunned, I sat speechless and smiling, looking down
at the engagement ring he once took off of my finger. I loved
him dearly, yet also feared his love was conditional.

"Let's make it forever this time," I said.

I knew that when Bryce felt pressure, he ran. He had
never been able to stay long enough to work through a
disagreement or let the dust settle after an argument. And
when he ran, he ran straight into the arms of another woman.

I was ridiculously happy yet also unsure if it was the
right thing for us. I loved Bryce, and I wanted so badly to
make things work. I simply surrendered to the idea that our
lives would unfold one day at a time as it was meant to. I

invited him to move in until we decided where to live. He decided to stay five nights at my house and two nights at his house since it was closer to where he worked.

~

As our pattern went, we lasted a mere two months. Lily Dale season was ramping up in June, and I had planned to assist Shirley with the Woman Empowerment Weekend. Bryce, on the other hand, wanted me to go on the Harley with him to a music festival. As usual, it led to a disagreement. I didn't want to give up my weekend event.

"I'm keeping my commitment to Shirley and the Woman Empowerment Weekend," I told him. "I signed up to attend months ago before we were even back together. I can't back out." Both of us were upset as I left my house. Driving the 20 minutes to Lily Dale, I knew he was packing and running again.

~

That night with Shirley and the other women attending was much needed. Shirley had become more than a teacher and mentor to me. I looked up to her as a mother figure. Before the class began, I confided in her my fears that Bryce would be gone when I got home.

Hugging me, she whispered so the others wouldn't hear, "Spirit is in control, Gail Lynn. Just keep asking for your highest and best… and breathe."

I sat for a while, teary-eyed. I had lost trust in Bryce, yet here I was wearing an engagement ring from him. Listening to Shirley speak to the women about loving oneself, I made a decision right then to do something different. I was not going to cry or be a victim anymore.

Shirley went around the circle allowing each woman to share insights or ask questions about what we had been learning with self-love. It was then that I heard a voice in my head again. When it was my turn to speak, tears welled up in my eyes.

"I am learning that I am important," I said. I took off the engagement ring and held it up. "I don't think the person who gave me this is ready for the commitment that comes with it. He is upset with me because I chose to be here instead of with him tonight at a music festival. I think he is at my house right now packing up his things. I know I need to learn to love myself more. I need to learn what love really is, and until then, I cannot wear this."

In my head, I saw visions of him packing his little black bag. I saw the dresser getting emptied. This odd feeling of *knowing* things was coming more frequently.

"I shouldn't have to worry whether my fiancé will be home when I get there or whether he will still love me if I go away for a weekend."

It was after 11:00 pm when I got home. I went straight to the bedroom and began opening the dresser drawers. As the visions showed me, they were empty. I stood there for a moment, staring at the void, feeling its message trying to take power over me.

Was I unlovable?

Instead of succumbing to the hurt and tears, I took a deep breath and walked out of the bedroom, closing the door behind me. Nothing warranted him leaving again. Going into the kitchen, I placed the engagement ring on the counter knowing he'd be back at some point to reclaim his ring.

I slept on the sofa that night feeling as empty as his drawer. It was an odd feeling. I didn't know which was worse, the emptiness or the yelling that was our other pattern.

The next morning, I pulled myself together and headed to Lily Dale for day two of the Woman Empowerment Weekend. One of the first activities was a breathwork meditation where we chose a partner, laid down on a mat one at a time, and were guided to hold space for the release of any fear, sadness, or trauma. Shirley suggested that instead of assisting her I work with a partner and do the exercise. I relinquished my need to be strong and allowed the memories of long-time trauma to emerge.

After that exercise, I felt another big release had occurred. Years of suppressed emotions were expelled. And I made some lifelong friends who became like sisters.

As Lily Dale opened for the season once again, I volunteered as a spiritual healer at The Healing Temple each day. As a workshop coordinator, I assisted all the presenters in their classes. I met many new people, and I came alive again. I worked on healing my heart and my life of abandonment and unworthiness. I learned about the metaphysical world that I had never known before.

The community of Lily Dale was a special world where I met world-renowned authors who had written books on science, philosophy, spiritualism, and healing. I interacted with people from all over the world and all walks of life. I began to step into new roles as a spiritual healer, as an intuitive and took classes to become an ordained minister.

I learned that as we grow and heal ourselves, we heal others. As we channel healing for others, we heal ourselves.

I was quite content and happy and again I had managed to pull myself back together after Bryce disappeared from my life. Again.

When the season ended Labor Day weekend, I spent that fall and winter engrossed in books, meditation classes, and spiritual development classes learning about this new world.

~

As Lily Dale season arrived in the summer of 2013, I helped with various classes. I assisted in a class on Emotional Freedom Technique (EFT) and then furthered that learning and became an EFT practitioner.

I learned more about mediumship and being a spiritual teacher as I assisted Lily Dale's spiritual teacher, healer, and retired registered medium, Dr. Judith Rochester.

Her class, "The Medium as the Teacher," encouraged me to begin creating my own workshops.

I continued to learn and practice mediumship with a spiritual teacher, Reverend Janet Nohavec, founder of The Journey Within School for Mediumship. In her class, "Evidential Mediumship," I began connecting with God, or as some say, Spirit, in a whole new way.

And then while assisting a class one day with Lily Dale medium, Reverend John White, I chuckled as he told me in a message, "One day you will write a book."

I was fascinated by John's abilities. In his workshop, "Remote Viewing," he was able to see into the homes of people in attendance. He gave evidence of their personal items that were inside the houses which he had never visited before.

I was happy. Life seemed to be improving for me, and I was truly following my bliss, or so it seemed.

Then the July 4th holiday approached, and I began rethinking Josh's accident and the breakup with Bryce. Scripts of the event replayed in my mind.

As our annual tradition went, I gathered the family to head to the 4th of July parade that morning. Happy to be sitting with James, Alycia, my grandkids, Josh, and Sara, I was elated. But then came the sirens blaring from the bright red firetrucks. Visions filled my mind of men in uniform knocking over chairs. The memories of the air raids that happened while skyping with my son during his time in Afghanistan were triggered. Then, as motorcycles drove by, I clutched my chest remembering the sight of Josh's motorcycle from his accident. I closed my eyes and plugged my ears. It didn't help. I stood and walked away so my kids wouldn't notice the tears welling up. My favorite holiday had become like a horror movie in my mind.

After getting through the parade, we headed back to my house for an afternoon of swimming and a barbeque. I tried to forget the events, so I grabbed a glass of wine and joined the kids in the pool.

Alycia was the first to mention fireworks. She knew my love for watching the magnificent colors light up the sky.

"James doesn't want to see fireworks, so he offered to take the kids back to the house so we can go," she said. "I think my brother and his buddy wants to ride with us too."

Later that evening, we found a spot to park at a restaurant on the lake, right where the fireworks were going to be let off. Getting out of the car, I heard the loud music coming from the deck of the restaurant. I recognized the singer's voice and knew it was a band that Bryce liked.

My heart raced at the thought of him being there. I quickly looked around the parking lot, but there was no sign of his truck. Then I scanned the crowd as we walked up on the deck, but there was no sight of him there either. I was relieved.

Alycia looked at the band and then over at me. She knew.

"Are you worried you might see Bryce?" she asked.

Shaking my head, "No." I lied.

"Good. Let's get a drink," she said cheerfully.

We headed to the bar and ordered. I kept looking around as if Bryce's ghost was peering over my shoulder. Something felt off, but I couldn't explain it. Extrasensory perception had become more refined. I kept looking over my shoulder as if he was going to simply appear. I kept having this feeling like something was going to happen, just like the night in my dining room two years before when I felt the same kind of odd feeling.

We got our drinks and headed to the dance floor. Loud music blared and brought back memories. Some were good, some not so much. Alycia began singing and suddenly grabbed my hand and began to twirl me around. I was grateful that she was here with me, grateful for my relationship with her.

"I love you," I said laughing. "Thanks for coming to see the fireworks with me."

"Of course! And I love you, too," she giggled. "I love watching the fireworks with you."

Then I saw him.

"He's here," I stammered.

Alycia looked around, and just as I was about to point, Bryce saw me. He quickly turned back to face the girl he was standing with. Then he leaned in and kissed her while watching me as if tempting me to react.

"Let's dance," Alycia said as she grabbed my arm.

"He's intentionally flaunting his relationship with this girl!" I shouted.

Not sure whether I was mad or sad, I closed my eyes and danced. I tried to erase the picture from my mind. I tried to close him out, but it wouldn't go away. All the memories came back in a flood. The weekend getaways and wine tasting, dancing, riding the Harley, and then the night he pulled the ring off my finger. I looked back to see where he was, but Alycia blocked my view.

"Why look at him?" she asked. "He's an idiot. Just have fun." She spun me around the dance floor again laughing.

"This is the man who professed his love for me, the man who proposed to me not just once but twice. We took trips together, made passionate love together, yet after every breakup, he runs to another woman. He doesn't know what love is."

We looked at him, and he looked at us. Grabbing her buttocks, he pulled his new girl in for a kiss all while watching me.

I was livid.

"You can't tell me that he's not intentionally trying to hurt me!" I shouted. "I'm going to tell him exactly what I think!"

"No, Gail," she held me back. "That's not a good idea. He's not worth your time. You're better than that. You *deserve* better than that. Think of all the times he hurt you and called you stupid. Think of the times when he betrayed your trust. And what about the times he got phone calls from other girls and hid it from you. Remember all the things about your relationship that did *not* work."

Alycia tried to steer me away from the line of vision, but I stood there, frozen, watching. Two years had passed, and I was still allowing him to hurt me. I stared at him as he smirked with some sort of sick pride in himself.

I broke down. I marched over to where he was standing against the bar and pushed my way in next to them as if bellying up to the bar. Then I turned and looked at the two of them.

"Oh! Hi, Bryce," I acted surprised to see him. Imagine seeing you here. Oh, that's right, you're one of the groupies who follow this band. How could I forget? That lead singer is right up your alley...trashy."

I turned and looked at the girl next to him.

"Hello," I sneered. "I'm Bryce's ex-fiancée. You must be his latest fling."

She looked at Bryce then back at me.

"Fiancée?" she snuffed. "You wish. Bryce's never been engaged."

"Oh, realllly?" The words rolled off my tongue in a southern drawl. "Well, as a matter of fact, he proposed *twice* in the past two years. And I was stupid enough to say yes both times. Isn't that right, Bryce?"

His eyes could have pierced holes right through me.

"Yeah, right," she said, turning to look at him for confirmation.

Elbowing me out of the way, he turned to his girl and said, "Don't listen to her."

"Really, Bryce? You're denying we were engaged? That you proposed to me, TWICE? We've been on and off for how many years now? Eight? Does your new girl here know you're a cheater? Does she know about that *other* thing, too?"

Vile words came spitting out of me.

"Be careful," I hissed. "He has a disease!"

I turned and walked towards Alycia, tears threatening to escape. It was time to go. I couldn't stomach another minute of being there. We found the rest of our group and left.

The little girl inside me cried out in pain.

WHY DID YOU LET HIM BACK IN?

I tried to hold back the tears. I scolded myself saying I should have behaved better, more spiritually, but my heart was in so much pain. Getting into the backseat of the car, I put my head between my legs trying to hide the shame, trying to silence the voice screaming in my head.

You'll never be good enough!

Shame, unworthiness, loneliness; these were the silent killers, like mysterious diseases that no doctor could treat.

How did you let him get under your skin?

~5~

My Initiation

Over the next two weeks, I teetered between wanting to hide, feeling ashamed of myself, and wanting to bathe in spiritual healing. Fortunately for me, my dad arrived from Phoenix to visit and took my attention elsewhere.

When he asked if I was interested in going on a road trip to New Jersey to visit relatives, I was glad to tag along. I needed something to keep my mind off of Bryce and the exchange we had.

It began as a wonderful adventure as Dad drove and I rode shotgun. My stepmom, Rosa insisted she sit in the back and that I take the front seat so that Dad and I could talk easier. She always encouraged us to be more open and communicate, knowing full well that Dad wasn't around much when I was growing up.

Arriving right about dinner time, I met my second cousins over a plate of barbequed spareribs, corn on the cob, and salad. Soon after we finished eating, one of them surprised Dad with a birthday cake and we all joined in singing happy birthday.

The following day we went to a big church to celebrate my cousin's 50th wedding anniversary. I met even more family over a buffet of food. Just as we were about to leave, we got invited to yet another cousin's house. With enough leftover food to feed the whole neighborhood, we gathered around the dinner table and continued to stuff ourselves with splendid food and Italian pastries.

Hearing a faint bark, I looked down to see a tiny teacup Pomeranian sitting at my feet. Reaching down, I scooped him up and placed him in my lap. I had never seen a dog so tiny or so adorable! Sitting cross-legged, he lay nestled in my lap for the next two hours until it was time for us to leave. Arriving back at my cousin's, I said goodnight and went straight to my room ready to turn in. Falling asleep, I thought of Bryce. A little voice inside me spoke, *I wonder if he is in love with the new girl now.*

~

The next day, everything changed.

It was July 23, 2013. The day the sickness in my body began.

Pain in my chest woke me in the early morning hours. I thought it was a dream. I thought a stranger was stabbing my chest with a fistful of daggers, but it was real.

I tried to sit up but couldn't move. I looked around to jog my memory. I was in New Jersey with my dad and Rosa staying with our relatives. A wave of panic crashed over me. The excruciating pain made me lightheaded. I thought I was going to die right there in my cousin's bed.

I moved my hands to my heart, then, closing my eyes, I prayed to God to take the pain away. Time seemed frozen as I laid there, and then I remembered the Reiki energy healing class that I had taken. In my mind, I used my finger to draw the Reiki symbols on my heart.

Just then, noises coming from the hallway caught my attention. *It must be my dad*, I thought. I tried to call out to him, but the pain took my breath away. I lay there for what felt like an eternity. Slowly, I managed to roll over and scooch my legs off the side of the bed. Sitting up, I clutched my chest and began rubbing where the pain was, but just as quickly as it had started, the pain dissipated.

I managed to get dressed and head downstairs. I heard voices coming from the kitchen, so I took a deep breath and made my way there.

"Good morning," all the voices chimed in.

The family was already engaged in conversations, coffee, and toast.

"How did you sleep?" asked my cousin.

"Fine, thank you," I said rather solemnly. I didn't want to worry anyone. "But I woke up with a little headache, though. Do you have any pain reliever?"

I took something for my headache and then poured a glass of orange juice. Rosa handed me a plate of bagels and a container of cream cheese. We made a plan to go to the ocean and walk, so I went back upstairs to get ready for our day and hoped the headache would go away. Going to the ocean was the only thing that moved me through the morning.

Within a short time, we were on our way.

I rode in the back seat of the car admiring the city views. The Statue of Liberty in the distance tugged at something in my heart. She looked so little, yet her energy was grand! This was where my dad and grandparents had arrived so many years ago as immigrants from Italy. My first glimpse of Lady Liberty came and went, and then, there it was. The Atlantic Ocean. It was a sunny, warm July morning. The sun's rays were creating blankets of diamonds across the sea. I was at peace, save for the headache.

As soon as the car was parked, I hopped out and ran to get a better view. I couldn't wait for everyone. I just wanted to put my feet in the sand. I turned and motioned for my family to hurry and catch up as I ran down to the water's edge. I felt the waves rushing over my feet. Surfers were catching small waves nearby, and it made me laugh to watch their novice attempts at riding the ocean.

Joy washed over me. I could have sat there in the sand and watched the sea all day, but my family called out to me to keep walking with them.

Back up on the boardwalk, little shops filled in the landscape along one side while views of the ocean still captured my attention on the other. It was my happy place.

We hadn't walked far when the morning's headache made its presence known again. I tried to ignore it, but the pain worsened, like someone bludgeoning me with a baseball bat.

As Dad and Rosa walked ahead, I soon lagged behind. Each step became more of an effort. I decided to head back down to the beach and put my feet in the sand. I thought the warmth of the sand would bring comfort. I was wrong. Every step became more torturous, and I had to stop every few feet and rest. With each step, excruciating pain shot up my foot, as if walking on shards of glass cutting me to the bone.

I had never experienced such agonizing pain before. Fearful of not being able to make it back to my family, I became overwhelmed with panic, and tears filled my eyes. Rosa saw me struggling and came to help.

"I don't know what's wrong," I shrieked. "Something's wrong with my feet, and the headache is back." I didn't want to cry. I hated crying. I hated feeling weak. Shivers ran up my spine recognizing the familiar energy that had returned.

The Fear Miser was back, I thought. Rosa took my arm and tried helping me, but I couldn't take another step. I sat down in the sand.

Rosa tried to comfort me, but there was nothing she could do or say to help alleviate the pain. She began waving her arms for my dad to see and catching his attention, he quickly came down to where we were.

"What happened?" he asked.

"I don't know, Daddy. My feet just started hurting and now I can barely walk."

"Come on, grab my arm. We'll walk up to the boardwalk to sit and have some lunch." My Italian family thought food could fix whatever ailed you. He helped me hobble to a pizzeria then ordered a bit of everything. When the food arrived, nothing looked good. I had no appetite. I was afraid. I didn't know what was wrong with me.

The family quickly ate then decided it was time to go. I hated the fact that I ruined the day. This was my happy place. The ocean, the sand, the sun. I couldn't enjoy any of it.

As we headed to the car, my body slowed to the pace of my 80-year-old grandmother. I was becoming fatigued and feeling feverish. Chills rippled through my body, and it wasn't The Fear Miser this time. It was something else. Something was very wrong.

~

The next day, Dad decided we should head back home to western New York. I agreed. I sat quietly in the car for eight hours wishing for sleep, but the pain I was feeling made it impossible.

When we got to my house, my father helped me inside. "You can leave, Daddy. I just want rest," I told him. "Sara should be home soon." I didn't know if that was true or not, but I just wanted to be alone. I was just so tired.

~

It was a restless night of profuse sweating. By morning, my sheets were soaked as if someone dumped a pan of water over me. Feeling chilled, I pulled the sheets up over me, but it hurt to have the sheets touch my legs. I pushed them off and laid there a while longer until it became too uncomfortable to even do that.

Tired and hungry, my thoughts were scattered. I eased my way out of bed and limped over to the stairs. I stood there staring at them as if they were a great mountain to climb. Instead, I sat down on the bottom step and then lifted my buttocks up to the next one and then the next, crawling my way up the stairs.

Feeling weak, I called out for Sara. I was hoping she made it home last night. It was early, so maybe she was still asleep and couldn't hear me. I called out again, but my voice crackled. I was sweating, trying to bear the pain, holding back the tears. Finally, I reached the top step, stood, and leaned up against the wall, and called out again.

"Sara!" I yelled. "Sara!" Sobs and tears took over me. The door creaked open, and she stepped out into the hallway looking sleepy and confused.

"I feel like I'm going to pass out," I told her. "I need to go to the doctor." Dizzy and nauseous, my body slowly melted onto the floor. It felt like I was leaving my body.

"Mom, what's wrong?" Sara rushed to my side.

"I don't know," I said. "The pain is so bad. I'm sorry, I need a doctor."

"What happened?"

"I don't know. I got sick while I was in New Jersey with Grandpa. I think I was bit by something. My sheets are soaked from sweating all night. I must have a fever. My body hurts. Look at my feet…." My voice trailed off and blended with the sobs that came bursting out.

"Oh my God, Mom, what can I do?" Sara stared in disbelief at my feet.

"Get your purse and help me to the car. I need a doctor."

Whimpering the 25 minutes to the local medical facility, I was hurting and afraid. I had no idea what was wrong.

Once inside, Sara explained to the receptionist my symptoms, and then a nurse appeared and asked us to follow her back into an exam room. Sara walked beside me, carrying the load of my weight.

"What brings you here today?" the nurse asked.

I told her about traveling to New Jersey, visiting with my family, and waking up in the morning with strong, fleeting chest pain. I mentioned the headache, the sharp pains in my feet, and not being able to walk. I filled her in about the few days beforehand leading up to this mysterious sickness.

"I was hiking through some woods last week and then bitten by mosquitos one night sitting by the lake. After that, I took a trip to New Jersey to visit my family. We were outside a lot. Maybe something bit me?" I asked inquisitively, tearing up again. "This morning I noticed this rash here by my ankle. It itches." She took my temperature and confirmed a fever.

The nurse recorded some things on her paper then opened the door just as the doctor appeared. He introduced himself and asked the same series of questions. Frustrated, I told the story once again. The trip, the lake, the rash. He glanced at my feet and commented on the inflammation.

"So, you've been doing a lot of walking?" he surmised.

"Yes," I responded. "And look here at this nodule thing on my leg. It started here on my wrist a couple of days ago then moved here to my leg yesterday."

He looked briefly at my leg then down at my flip-flops on the floor. "Are those the shoes that you wear when you walk?" he asked.

"Yes," I said. "I wear flip-flops during the summer."

"Are these the shoes you wore when you were hiking also?"

"Yes." Changing the subject back to my symptoms, I asked him. "Do you think my symptoms could be related to the West Nile virus that has been in the news?"

"Did you wear these flats on your trip, too?"

"Yes! But the pain throughout my body isn't about my *shoes*. What about the rash? The mosquito bites? The fever and chills? The sweating at night? The insomnia? These don't have anything to do with my shoes!"

"It appears you have Plantar Fasciitis," he said dismissively. "I'll give you a prescription for the pain, but you should follow up with your primary care doctor next week."

"What is Plantar Fasciitis?" I asked.

"The answer to your problem is to get different shoes. A woman your age should be wearing supportive shoes."

I shot Sara a look then turned back to him in disgust. He wrote up a prescription and handed it to me.

"I think I was bitten by something," I said angrily. "This is *not* from wearing flip-flops."

He just walked away and told me to follow-up with my primary care doctor on Monday...and to buy supportive shoes.

I turned to look at Sara. "What the hell are supportive shoes? Is he serious?" I yelled out the door, not caring who heard me. "He's blaming this all on flip-flops?"

"Come on, Mom," she said. "Let's just go get your prescription. Are you hungry? We'll stop and get some of your favorite soup."

I wasn't hungry. I was defeated, and the doctor was of no help.

We drove silently to the pharmacy then home. Having Sara at my side was the only thing keeping me from losing my sanity. I could see the concern on her face as we struggled to the sofa. I laid back on the pillow and without another word, she went and fetched a blanket to cover me. I was shaking with chills and sweating profusely again.

I tried to get comfortable, but it was impossible. I pushed the blanket off my legs and rolled to my side. That hurt worse. I tried to elevate my legs on a pillow, but that didn't help. There was no way to relax, so I stood and headed to the kitchen instead.

"What do you need, Mom?" she asked. "Let me help you. Are you hungry? Want some soup?"

I didn't know what I needed. I paced back and forth until she came over and put her arms around me as I cried.

We stood there in the middle of the kitchen, my baby girl soothing her mother. After a few minutes, she walked me back to the sofa.

I put my legs up on the coffee table with a soft pillow supporting my ankles. "Look at them," I said pointing. My legs and ankles were thick and swollen. "I look like I have elephant legs." Sara laughed. Sometimes, the only way to deal with the pain in life was to find something to laugh about.

Sara reached for the remote and turned on the television. I laid my head back on a pillow and closed my eyes. As hours passed, the pain worsened, the fever and chills persisted. The comfort of a blanket that I normally sought only increased the pain. It hurt to stand. It hurt to sit. It hurt to lay down. It hurt to breathe. I had never known pain like that before, not even when I gave birth to my children.

Let me die, I thought.

~

The next week, I followed up with my family doctor, but it only brought more confusion and a different diagnosis.

"I think you have gout," the doctor's assistant said. "I want to run some blood tests and see you back here next week. I want the doctor to get a look at you, too."

I begged for help to relieve the pain, so the assistant checked with the doctor and they agreed to change my pain medication to something a little stronger.

"I don't normally take medicine," I informed her. "Not even an aspirin for a headache. Why isn't this pain medication working?" She simply shrugged her shoulders and said she'd get back to me with the results of the blood work.

Later that day, vials of blood were taken, tests for numerous diseases were done, and all of the results were inconclusive. A few weeks later, another change in medication and more blood tests led to another attempt at a diagnosis.

"I believe it could be Lupus," said the doctor during another visit. But again, after more bloodwork, that was ruled out as well.

"This is really a mystery," the doctor said on the phone one day. I want to refer you to a specialist for Rheumatoid Arthritis." I felt like a guinea pig, a science experiment for doctors to practice on.

Meanwhile, a toothache started along with a tingling sensation in my head. The nodules that kept appearing on my body looked like aliens invading and moving from one location to another. They appeared one day as a large red lump, turned black and blue, then disappeared only to reappear in a different location on my body. One day on my leg, another day on my wrist, a day or two later it showed up on my knee. All the while, insomnia had set in and brain fog had kept me from thinking or speaking clearly. The buzzing beehive in my head just kept getting worse.

People in my church began to pray for me. On the occasion that I felt strong enough, I drove myself to The Healing Temple in Lily Dale. Sitting on a bench with a healer standing behind me, I cried. Sundays I limped my way up the church stairs to sit on a bench for healing while community members prayed over me. Nothing took the pain away.

I began asking over and over, *God, what did I do to deserve this?*

~

Each day brought on new symptoms, and having any kind of life was just about impossible. Frustrated, I was determined to do something normal. So, I called my friend, Darlene, and asked her to meet me at the coffee shop in the local grocery store. The 20-minute drive was not the best idea. Leaving my house, I felt normal, but somewhere along the way, I forgot where I was going.

"Where am I?" I panicked.

Stopped at a traffic light, I didn't know which way to go. I pulled over into a parking area and sat there afraid and confused. I felt like a little child lost and wanting her mommy.

I reached for my cell phone to look through the contacts and found "Mom" then pressed the call icon.

"Hi, sweetie," she answered. Her familiar voice comforted me. Without telling her what was wrong, we conversed long enough for me to remember that I was heading to the grocery store in my hometown and meeting my friend, Darlene. We chatted until I gained my confidence back, and then I continued on to the store, Mom being none the wiser.

"You look awful," Dar said when she caught sight of me. "You look like an 80-year-old. I didn't recognize you."

"Thank you," I said. "I love you, too." We laughed, and that was enough to hide my fear.

Over lunch, I shared my story with her about the struggles and symptoms and various doctors. "You don't know what's causing this?" she asked.

"No. And the doctors don't know either. It's a mystery."

~

Life went on around me as summer came to an end. School would be starting up again soon and I had to figure out what to do about returning to my classroom. I didn't know if I could go back to teaching. I often forgot where I was driving and didn't know how safe it was to commute half an hour each day to and from school. I was fatigued most of the time. I didn't know if I could stand in front of 20 young children and do my job well. The doctors couldn't tell me what was wrong. No one had answers to the pain or beehive tingling in my head or the mysterious nodules growing on my body. I felt like a lost soul.

While doctors gave me one diagnosis after another, I began seeking answers myself. I went to various spiritual healers in the community and sought the advice of new thought leaders and energy healers who came to Lily Dale.

On one occasion, I sat in a class taught by actress and spiritual healer, Dee Wallace. She placed me in the center of the room and asked everyone to join together and simultaneously send me healing. I felt better for a few hours. On another occasion, I talked briefly with the author, Neale Donald Walsch, after his presentation in my community and asked him for prayers as well. I was grasping for help.

Weeks and weeks of doctor's appointments came and went. My job at the elementary school was put on hold. I spent most of my time alone staring at walls or pacing the floors or sleeping. When I felt up to the task, I began to research my symptoms online. I typed in: "What causes inflammation and how to reduce it" and "How to improve gut health to reduce inflammation" and "West Nile Virus and other diseases from mosquitos."

I spent hours conversing with Spirit, but it felt one-sided. Even when I heard answers, I was sure that they were only coming from the confines of my own mind, and I surely did not trust the source of such thoughts.

Each week that passed seemed to bring more symptoms and more pain. Each doctor and test and medication seemed useless. Each misdiagnosis brought greater despair. The Lupus specialists, Rheumatoid Arthritis specialist, a world-renowned clinic, spiritual healers, and energy workers were all stumped as to how to help me get well. I looked for answers everywhere.

Finally, a friend invited me to a medical séance in Lily Dale. I attended, of course, and as the evening ended, the medical intuitive who was doing the séance told me what I needed to hear.

"We think you may have Lyme disease," she said.

"What is Lyme disease?" I asked.

"Lyme disease is a very smart bacteria, often called the great imitator, as it mimics so many different illnesses," said the woman. "It can appear as chronic fatigue, fibromyalgia, arthritis, lupus, Parkinson's, Lou Gehrig's, multiple sclerosis, and more. The bacteria, called a spirochete, can invade every organ of the body, including the heart, lungs, into the central nervous system, and the brain."

The medical intuitive made some suggestions for me to begin to address the symptoms. A few hundred dollars later, my counter was covered with supplements of various colors, shapes, and sizes. The herbal supplements blended right in with the antibiotics and pain killers from the doctors. Sadly, my counter looked like a pharmacy. At the very least, I had a new diagnosis to look into.

During my endless nights of insomnia, I began to research Lyme disease. I wanted to know how I got it, why I got it, where it came from, what I could do to get rid of it, and when it started. I began to gather information and collect my own evidence of what was going on with my body.

I started to wonder if it began that night in Lily Dale when I sat by the lake and was bitten by mosquitos. Or if it happened during the road trip with my father to New Jersey. I even considered an idea a local friend told me, that it was a hex put on me by a jealous neighbor. None of it mattered though. What I wanted to know most of all was how to heal from this mysterious sickness that had gotten inside me.

The symptoms were too numerous for the average person to understand. Trying to explain what it was like to have this God-awful illness was nearly impossible. *Dis*-ease in the body was affecting every cell, organ, nerve, and tissue of mine. The brain fog made me some combination of a child with ADHD and autism coupled with an elderly person with the beginning stages of Alzheimer's.

Conducting my own research, I began to learn ways to ease inflammation through diet. I immediately eliminated all meat, dairy, and store-bought foods put in cans, boxes, packages, and containers. I ate only live and organic food from the produce section of the grocery store. I made green smoothies for breakfast and lunch every day. For dinner, I ate salads and other vegetables. I made bone broth soup. Eating properly became my full-time job.

It was late one night with insomnia when I found the documentary, *Under Our Skin*. Five minutes into it, I sat up in bed with new vigor. Others were experiencing this same thing. I wasn't crazy. I had made a connection with others.

Still, I asked God, *Why did this happen?*

As I watched and learned about the hidden epidemic of Lyme disease and how the health care system was failing to address it, the comfort of knowing WHAT I had did not soothe the question WHY I had it. It broke my heart as I watched the documentary again.

As I learned more about Lyme disease, I came across many stories as to where it all began. Controversy surrounded this disease.

I didn't know what to believe.

~6~

Who Do I Trust?

Discerning truth can be difficult, and given the amount of stress and suffering I was experiencing, knowing what to believe or even WHO to believe made life even more challenging. Even the top experts in their field disagreed on diagnosis and treatment, and I lost faith in the medical system.

Because my doctor felt I wasn't strong enough to return to my job teaching in September, I spent many restless days home and alone, feeling sorry for myself. New symptoms emerged each week and wreaked havoc on my body, and I questioned why.

Each day blended with the next. Sitting on the sofa with my laptop, I went from one website to another trying to find answers. Some days I prayed, some days I looked up at the ceiling and yelled with fury through my tears.

"Hello... are you real? If you are, why aren't you helping me?" I began questioning this God I was taught about and if "He" was really there listening to our prayers.

After forcing myself out of bed each morning, I would head to the kitchen to start my day. Walking back and forth from the refrigerator to the sink, I got out green apples, cucumbers, and carrots. I washed them off, cut them into chunks to fit into my Vitamix, and then added in a handful of fresh organic spinach or kale. Adding frozen fruit and then finally coconut water, I blended it for my morning meal.

A good chunk of every morning was spent like this, washing and cutting up fresh fruit and vegetables to have a meal my stomach could handle. Like most of the symptoms, nausea came and went, and I never knew if it was going to be a good day that I would spend sitting on the sofa or patio researching OR a day spent in bed.

Monotony is an evil companion that threatens well-being just as loneliness does.

Weeks passed with no progress. Then, on a rare occasion, something would arise that gave me a ray of hope, like the few occasions when my daughter was able to come home from college. Her company was a ray of sunshine in my dismal life. Mostly though, the days were filled with pain and fear. I questioned my existence. In all honesty, I wanted to die.

Sometimes I made it a game to challenge myself to do something "normal." Although I feared getting lost again, getting out of the house was a necessity. One morning I woke up and wanted to be near the water. I wanted to put my feet in the sand and watch the waves crash onto the shore. I drove to the local beach. It was my happy place.

It was a bright and sunny September day. At first, I was glad. No screaming kids or parents yelling, just serenity. After about 20 minutes of sitting and admiring the sun dance upon the water, the solitude turned to loneliness. I started to think about my colleagues in their classrooms. Then I thought about my own classroom of students and felt an overwhelming sadness. Someone else had taken my place. Someone else was doing my job, teaching my students, reading with them, doing math problems with them, and talking with them about how to be good citizens. The peace quickly turned to despair as these thoughts entered my head, so I left.

I drove home and sat on my sofa and cried. I wanted to go back to my classroom and be the one making a difference in their lives, but I couldn't. What hurt me the most was that my colleagues didn't understand. Several of them joked about "the good life" I had. Being home every day made them jealous. They didn't understand the pain or loneliness I felt. Their perception of my life made them envious, whereas I yearned to have theirs.

After that day at the beach, I decided to put all of my effort and energy into figuring out this illness. Every day I sought answers from spiritual healers and doctors to better understand why this happened to me. I went from doctor to naturopath to an energy healer. I went to a few yoga classes and a chiropractor and then a nutritionist and an acupuncturist, but no one had the answer.

Weeks turned to months, and I got an appointment at a world-renowned clinic. Seventeen vials of blood later, as I was being pushed out in a wheelchair, I was told that my white blood cell count was improving in comparison to previous tests.

"Whatever you're doing, keep doing it," was the advice from one of the doctors.

I guess I was expecting more. I was expecting answers, a diagnosis, a reason, or at the very least a direction to take or some advice about what to do next. But there wasn't any of that, nor did I feel any better. The medical system let me down, again. I was angry at the medical world. Even they abandoned me.

My friend, Patsy, who had accompanied me to the appointment, tried to make me feel better. She invited me to stay overnight and took me to dinner at a beautiful restaurant overlooking Lake Erie. On our walk from the car to the door, I felt like I was walking on thumbtacks. I thought that if I went slower, the pain wouldn't be so bad, but I was wrong. I winced with every step, and she walked right there beside me. I was thankful for her. After dinner, we made our way down to the lake. I needed to be near the water.

Later that evening, we talked about how the author's in the spiritual world handle illness, most often looking at emotions stuck in the body and using some form of energy work to heal.

The following day, I decided to stop at a bookstore on my way home and purchase a few metaphysical self-help books that my friend had recommended. I wanted to immerse myself more fully in these spiritual teachings.

I began to read over and over again this idea that thoughts create things. I read the work of the author, Louise Hay, and adopted her outlook that when our thoughts are not positive or not aligned with a higher vibration, we can become ill. Chapter by chapter, I read how certain negative thoughts could lead to specific illnesses, and different sicknesses correlated with a specific area of the physical body.

I began to pay attention to this in my own world. I listened to the people around me to see how this would work, to see how it actually fits into a person's experience. I looked at my own life and considered how this related to the Lyme disease, if at all. I questioned myself as to whether I did something to create the illness in my body, whether my thoughts had created the disease in me. It stretched my beliefs, but I was willing to consider it.

~

The following day I received a call from a girl I had met at the coffee shop in Lily Dale.

"Hi, Gail. This is Brenda," she reintroduced herself. "We met in Lily Dale. I heard someone say you may have Lyme disease. I have it, too. I go to a Lyme literate specialist a few hours away." She gave me his number and wished me well.

I had hope again.

I called immediately and made an appointment for the following month. Still not back to teaching, my daily goal was simply to get through the day with enough energy to do basic tasks of showering, making meals (smoothies), and doing laundry. Symptoms varied extensively. Some days I was so fatigued that watching the television was exhausting. Other days the pain was so bad I couldn't sit, walk, or sleep without wincing from sharp stabbing pains in my legs. Those were the worst days. I didn't know what to do with myself.

My primary care doctor still had me on and off amoxicillin and pain medications, but nothing helped any of the symptoms disappear. Bright lights hurt my eyes, loud noises hurt my ears, and a constant buzzing in my head contributed to anxiety that settled in me every single day.

Being home alone all the time didn't help. I was grateful when my friend from high school, Jen, called and invited me to visit her in Virginia. The Fear Miser threatened that I couldn't drive that far, but again, I made a game out of it and threw caution to the wind. I called my mom and told her my plan to drive south. I asked her to call and check on me in an hour. Then I threw a bunch of clothes into a small travel bag and headed out the door. I was determined to be "normal" as I rolled down the windows, turned up the music, and forgot my world of sickness for a while.

The seven hours in the car went by quickly. First Mom called and we chatted for a good two hours. And then Darlene called. I was grateful for both of their company. I arrived around dinnertime, and Jen welcomed me with excitement. The weekend visit turned out to be a weeklong stay when she decided a side trip to Virginia Beach would be good for me.

The sunshine and laughter with my friend were healing. We floated in the ocean all day.

"God will take care of you," she reminded me.

A week later, it was time to return home. The Fear Miser made an appearance to remind me of what I had to look forward to: loneliness, sickness, confusion, and unanswered prayers. And then I began to wonder.

Why did I feel better when I was with Jen? Was it the sunshine or laughter or the minerals in the ocean water that eased my symptoms?

The closer I got to home, the more my energy level diminished.

~

The week after I got home was my long-awaited doctor's appointment. When I arrived in Doctor Munshi's office, I was greeted and handed a ten-page checklist of symptoms[1] to read through. I was to note each symptom that I had experienced with a checkmark. As I sat in the waiting room flipping page after page, the pen was afire with marking each symptom. Joint pain, bone sensitivity, tendonitis, chronic fatigue. Yes, yes, yes, yes. It was unbelievable how many symptoms were associated with Lyme disease. Overwhelmed, I cried in that cold waiting room as I sat alone. I wondered yet again what I had done to deserve this.

On that first visit, the doctor did an EKG test, a neurological exam, some observation of sensory-motor movements, and then we discussed my symptoms.

"You have Lyme disease," he concluded, then went on to explain that there was a blood test offered by a specific lab that he wanted me to complete to distinguish which co-infections I had as well. He told me about the difficulties that came with Lyme disease, the host of co-infections, and how every day can bring a multitude of new symptoms. He explained how the bacteria infiltrates every part of the body making it necessary to rest, eat well, stay hydrated, and avoid stress. He told me I would be off of work for a while and handed me a prescription for a 30-day supply of doxycycline. I was to make an appointment to be seen again after the doxy was completed.

---

[1] For a reference list of symptoms see Appendix A

"You need to focus on your health," he warned. "Stop worrying about your job. Stress kills people. You need to rebuild your immune system."

Those words frightened me as he sat staring at his papers. Then he took my hand in his as he began looking at my fingernails. Watching him, something changed in his face.

"You're not a doctor," I said as I gazed into his eyes. He suddenly felt familiar, like I had known him from somewhere.

"Of course I'm a doctor!" he smiled. "What do you mean?"

"You're a healer," I whispered. "I trust you. Where are you from?"

He turned to look at me and smiled again. Pointing to a map on the wall. "India," he responded.

I nodded already knowing that he was going to say India. That was how I knew him, but I couldn't explain it.

"I knew that," I said. Then, changing the subject, I asked him, "When will I be better?"

He simply shrugged his shoulders. "We shall see."

~

Back home, I felt relieved. I had hope again. I was determined to get better and started to look for the next trick to add to my bag of tools. I spent hours on the internet searching Lyme communities to see what had worked for others. Some people found relief in using an infrared sauna and dry skin brushing. I also found research on a technique called Earthing and incorporated that into my regimen as well. I was hungry for healing.

My doctor was treating me with doxycycline, and I was on the prayer list of several local churches. I was attending meditation classes when I felt up to driving and sitting for spiritual healing in my church on Sunday mornings. I felt comforted.

Day after day, I contemplated my life. Day after day, I continued to seek healing. I removed things from my life that I had read were not good for my body. I tossed out all my toothpaste with fluoride and body creams with toxic chemicals. I eliminated everything that didn't feel right on my healing journey. My intuition became stronger, and oftentimes, I just *knew* what was good for me and what wasn't.

As I eliminated what wasn't good for me, I began to feel better and stronger. That's when the urge began. I longed to work and have my normal life back again.

The thought of going back to work was scary, but I was up for it. Four months after becoming ill, I finally had the courage to try teaching again. At my doctor's appointment, I told him I wanted to try.

"It will be a tough transition," Doc Munshi said contemplatively. "Are you sure you're ready? Will your school support you?"

He was right to question my decision. To go from no responsibilities at home for the past four months to all the demands of teaching and being back at school was no small change. There were strict schedules and 20 high energy kids. There were lesson plans, emails, meetings, testing, data input, and a whole slew of responsibilities that came with being an elementary school teacher. It could be too much all at once. The thought was scary, but living life as I was, was scarier.

Doc Munshi shared his concern and suggested that I only work half days. He cleared me to return to work, part-time. I would use the mornings to prepare myself. I would start back in the afternoons for my first three days. The school administration supported the idea that both my students and I should ease in slowly through the transition.

In preparation for what was to come, I began to "practice" my mornings. I set my alarm for 6:00 am every day as if I was going to work. I went through the routine of showering, getting dressed, and making breakfast as if I was going to head out the door at the designated time to get to my classroom on time.

It was an odd feeling to practice my life, but it was needed. It was not an easy feat to do these things. Some mornings I had to force myself out of bed even when my body was too exhausted and refusing to cooperate, but I pushed myself. I trusted life was going to support me. I trusted the school would support me. I trusted God and the angels would support me.

~7~

Conflicts & Obstacles

When the day finally arrived that I could return to work, I awoke from a bad dream about entering a lion's den. The Fear Miser was back. I remembered the first time the new principal walked into my classroom and humiliated me in front of my students. The thought kept haunting me like a ghost from the past that wouldn't leave. I tried to shake it off. I tried thinking of the new students who were eagerly waiting to meet me, but then another thought entered. The Fear Miser was having fun with me.

A colleague called and said every one of my substitutes left school angry each day. The children in my classroom were causing disruptions to the point where many of the subs never returned.

"The principal changed the class lists before school started. You have all the students with behavioral problems. She is hoping you will quit," my colleague informed me.

I shook the memory of that dreaded conversation out of my head. With my jar of green smoothie in hand, I headed out the door. My intention was to pray my way to work, but what happened instead was that thoughts were on repeat of all the unpleasant interactions that had occurred between me and the principal.

When I walked into my classroom that morning, the young substitute looked happy to see me. She seemed ready and eager to hand my students over. She explained with trepidation why the big red bouncy ball was being passed around the room by some of the boys. "I read an article that suggested boys needed more opportunities to release their energy," she said. "I thought my yoga ball would help."

It was chaos, but I felt nothing but sympathy. The principal introduced us and laughed at the boys bouncing on the ball, then she introduced me to the class as their *real* teacher.

"Oh! Ms. Gail!" one of the boys sang out. "I'm so glad you're back! We didn't think you'd ever get here. We heard you were sick."

The children ran up to me, and I was suddenly immersed in a mob of eight-year-olds all joining arms around me in a group hug. Losing my balance, I stepped back as several of them stuck papers in my face shouting, "We made cards for you!"

My heart melted at their kindness. Being the center of attention for that brief moment was a delight. Tears welled up in my eyes and then one of the girls noticed.

"Hey, guys," she said, "give Ms. Gail some room, you're hurting her. Ms. Gail, come over here, sit on the carpet. We'll hand you the cards one at a time." She spoke so kindly.

I looked over at the principal as she turned and walked away. Having the sub there as an extra set of hands and eyes would be helpful as I learned about my students and adjusted the routines. I followed the kids to the carpet and began to read their letters. Kindness flowed from their words as did their fears of being unable to read well or do math. When I finished reading the last letter, I looked up at my students.

"You are now my students," I said, "MY children, and I will do everything I can to help you succeed."

An hour passed before the phone rang. It was the principal. She asked to speak to the sub.

Handing her the phone, I stood by and waited to see if the principal wanted to talk to me again. She looked uneasy as she nodded and repeated, "Uh-huh, okay," and all the while her eyes were on me. After she hung up, she told me she had to go to the office.

"They need me to make copies," she said. "They have some letters that need to go home before the end of the day."

I was confused. "Really? You were supposed to be in the classroom with me all afternoon."

"I'm sorry. I'm just... I have to follow directions." She turned and walked out the door.

Determined not to let this little misunderstanding or The Fear Miser get to me, I turned back to my students and smiled.

"Looks like I get you all to myself!"

The school day wrapped up and the sub finally walked back into the classroom. She looked a little uneasy as she gathered up her belongings. I interrupted the frenzy.

"We need to go over the lesson plans for the week. Can you show me where you have them?"

"I can't stay," she said, putting on her jacket. "I have someplace I have to be."

"Are you okay?" I asked. "Is something wrong?

"I have to get to an appointment," she said.

"Okay, but where are the lesson plans?" She was to have the weekly lesson plans completed last Friday and on the desk for the administrator's review. I was confused. I began to sense something was wrong,

She kept her head down and avoided eye contact.

"Is everything okay?" I asked again.

She looked around as if to see if anyone was in the room. "I was told not to help you," she whispered. "The principal told me to leave right at 3:00 pm when the students leave. She told me not to walk your students to gym or library or lunch. She said that you're supposed to do that. I'm sorry."

The next day was the same. When I arrived for the afternoon, the substitute left for other duties that the office needed help with. There were no lesson plans for the afternoon, only some unexplained notes of activities that she had done in the morning. When she came back at the end of the day, I asked for clarification.

"Have you done testing to put the students in reading groups yet? What unit are you in for math?"

She struggled to answer. "I haven't done reading groups. The principal said you would do it when you returned. As for math, the other teachers have been giving me copies of their worksheets. There have been so many substitutes, it was kind of a mess when I started." As she left, I thanked her for working with my students and not quitting on them.

~

I began moving desks around. I put up a new bulletin board for reading and writing groups and then made another for behavior expectations. I stopped trying to figure out what lessons she had taught in the curriculum and instead created some activities for my students that could show me their writing skills. I pulled out testing material so I could begin to form reading groups. Two months behind, I had a lot to do to get the students caught up.

My students didn't like the new expectations and began acting out even more. When I picked them up from library class, the librarian made a loud comment for us all to hear as we left.

"I don't know how you do it, Ms. Gail. I had to separate six of your students today." I could see the frustration on her face.

"I'm sorry," I sighed. "They'll do better next time."

As we slowly reentered the classroom, I whispered to my students that we would have a few minutes of quiet time to think about what happened in the library. I set a timer for three minutes, and when the timer went off, I began to call the students one by one to join me on the carpet.

"Let's talk," I said. "Who wants to start?"

Each one had an opportunity to speak. They shared stories about their frustration with math or reading. They talked about their home life and how other students were noisy and kept them from learning. It was exhausting, but I needed to listen. I needed to create an environment where they felt safe and nurtured and where they knew what was expected of them. Otherwise, the behaviors would continue. I wanted them to have tools to use to deal with their frustrations or anger, so together we came up with a plan.

Getting two extra desks for the room, we decided to put one desk next to mine and the other in a corner by itself.

"We will give this a try," I told my students. "If you need quiet time to yourself, you have permission to get up and sit at either desk if you need a break." Some of them used the desks effectively, some of them used it to avoid doing their work, but it was especially helpful for those who wanted a quiet area away from the noise to get their work done.

It was normal to have seven or eight students acting out all at the same time. Finally, I decided to go to the office and read their personal folders and reports from previous teachers. Eight of my students had files containing notes with comments: incorrigible, lacking motivation, downright mean, or violent to other students and staff.

Reading further about the home life and family situations, my heart broke for many of them. One child lived with a relative because the parents were in jail. Another shared a bedroom with four siblings. Another was visited by a previous teacher and the home was found to have no beds at all.

Each day, behaviors in the classroom worsened as the honeymoon period ended. Students were no longer happy as I pushed them to complete work and do their best. On top of it all, the principal often popped her head in, smirking as if pleased with my struggles.

One day, her comment pushed the wrong button as she stepped inside the room and watched us play a game of hangman. Little did she know the words were pulled from their latest writing assignment.

"I hope you're teaching the common core and not just playing games," she said. "Your students need to catch up."

Inciting me to anger, I finally spat back.

"Did you ever check to see what the substitute taught? She had no lesson plans and no reading groups. I *am* catching my students up, but many of them also need to learn how to get along in a classroom." I stomped away like an angry child.

Needless to say, she walked out, calling out over her shoulder, "I want to see your lesson plans first thing tomorrow. They are behind because of *you*."

"Sure," I stated.

Returning to the front of the classroom to write another sentence on the board, the students sat and stared at me. They had heard the whole exchange and were now sitting in silence, drawing their own conclusions.

That night I spent hours creating a new schedule. Minute by minute, I planned out lessons for the next week. I left no room for the sweet, teachable moments that I loved, but instead, I crammed in lesson after lesson to please the principal. After preparing activities for five different reading groups and four different math groups, I fell asleep exhausted and worried, wondering if it would be enough for her.

As directed, I had my lesson plans available for her to see the next day. She stopped in during my morning math lesson, went to my desk, and looked at my plans. She wrote on a sticky note, then walked out. I went over to read it.

"Looks Good."

Yes, pretty, I thought. Like I don't know how to teach? After eighteen years and many administrators and teachers requesting their child to be in my classroom, being targeted in this manner was demeaning. I had been in the newspaper for the curriculum that I wrote and taught. I had many students reach the highest level on the state exam. I even went back to night school to get my administrative certification to step into the role of principal one day. THIS was not good leadership. I sat and gave myself a pity party while my students solved their multiplication problems.

~

When the weekend finally arrived, I stayed in my pajamas, read a little, then Darlene called.

"We're making plans for the annual Disco," she said. "You're going to come, aren't you?"

Great. *Another thing I can't do*, I thought. "Of course not, Dar, I can barely walk let alone stand on my feet all night or dance."

"Jerry and I already talked. You can stay in the room with my daughter. There's plenty of room. I'm going to my brother's house tomorrow to get an old wheelchair. Jerry said he would push you in the wheelchair so that you didn't have to walk and so you'd have a place to sit all night."

Wonderful, I thought. Sitting in a wheelchair all night while everyone around me was dancing.

My heart was heavy at the thought of missing the night of fun with my friends. I wanted to go laugh and dance and be silly, but life was full of conflicts now, and this was just one more obstacle to overcome.

"You're not going to sit home in self-pity. We're picking you up, bringing you to your room, pushing you down the streets of Buffalo and into that disco!" Darlene was adamant that I was going with them. "We WILL have fun, just like always!"

She didn't understand, but I agreed to go.

As the night of the disco began, I already felt out of place. Jerry parked in front of the hotel, and we got out. Darlene grabbed our bags while Jerry opened the trunk and pulled out the wheelchair. My heart sank. Despising its existence, I wanted to pick it up and throw it. Looking at the cold steel armrests and the brown plastic seat, the sudden realization hit me. I needed a wheelchair to go to the disco.

Darlene looked at me and then at the wheelchair.

"Don't look like that," she smiled at me. "See what I brought? Glitter! We're going to get this thing all jazzed up for you. I know you like sparkles, so we will spray this glitter paint on and make it pretty!"

"Dar," I forced a laugh as I teared up. Only she would think to bring glitter. "What would I do without you?"

"Stop," she teased. "You're going to make me cry, and we're not going to do that. We're going to have fun tonight just like we always do." She hugged me

"I love you, Dar," I said. "Thank you. And Jerry, thank you for being here to help and for being willing to push me down the streets of Buffalo in this... this thing." I sat down in the wheelchair and Jerry pushed me to my room, which connected right to theirs.

A short while later, the rest of our friends arrived. Dar made us each a cocktail and we toasted to the evening. Dar grabbed her camera for our usual picture taking frenzy, but I told her, "No. I don't want to be in any of the photos this year, though. I feel ugly. I don't want to capture any of these moments. I hate this new version of myself."

Looking into the mirror, I heard that inner critic, *You're despicable. Go away. Bring back the old Gail.*

She pretended she didn't hear me. "Come on Gail, get over here. Jerry's going to take our picture."

I put on a fake smile, the one everyone wanted to see, the one I wore all my years while growing up.

Then the girls began to take turns sitting in the wheelchair and making it seem less horrible.

"I'm going to want a turn in this tonight!" said one.

94

"This is a good thing to have with us!" said another.

"It's comfy!"

"Give it a try," they said to Dar.

I would have laughed with them if it wasn't I who had to rely on it. I wanted my life back. It took all I had not to scream at them. I wanted them to stop laughing, to stop making fun. A smile covered up my wish to disappear.

The rest of the evening was the same sort of mood. Being pushed down the city streets in a wheelchair while people stared at me with pity was heart-wrenching. The World's Largest Disco was an annual highlight for us, but watching thousands of people dancing and not being able to participate was not my kind of fun. After a few hours, one of the girls pulled me up to dance and tried to twirl me around while another sat in the wheelchair happy to be off her feet. Whenever one of them looked my way, I smiled.

As planned, Jerry returned at midnight, pushed me back down the cold city streets of Buffalo on that November evening with the rest of the girls trailing behind. He wheeled me back to the hotel, back to my reality.

I was sick. My life force had left me.

~

Weeks went by, and I knew a setback was coming. The daily stress and conflicts with students and the principal finally caught up to me. I took a day off to go see my doctor.

"What is going on?" he asked. "How are you feeling?"

"Work is very stressful. The principal is still nitpicking everything I do. I think she tries to make every day difficult for me on purpose. Day after day, week after week...she's relentless. She hates me. I'm tired of it all." The tears came. "I just want my life back."

He looked down at my hands in quiet contemplation. "You have two choices," he said. "Either quit and get your health back or keep going and allow the stress to build up.

95

Are you drinking enough water? The last tests we did show that you have antibodies for gluten intolerance. The number is high. Any gluten will only make your health worse. You have Celiac Disease. You have to stop eating anything with gluten."

Frowning with disappointment, I asked him, "What's Celiac Disease?" *Another diagnosis, another obstacle, and more to research*, I thought.

"The nurse will give you some handouts on Celiac Disease when you check out. You have to avoid the stress. Stress can kill you. It is what causes the flareups." He handed me a script for more bloodwork and told me to make another appointment after the bloodwork was done.

My day off of work was spent driving almost three hours to see Doc Munshi and then three hours back. No time to rest. The following day I was back in the classroom with students who were happy to see me again. They told me they thought I was going to be gone for a long time again. Some of them had even made another card for me.

"Get well soon, Ms. Gail!" one card said. "I hope I didn't make you sick." They clamored around me and gave me the notes and cards they had made. I was enjoying their compassion until I heard footsteps and looked up to see the principal.

"Glad you're back today," she sneered. "I'm here to see your lesson plans."

"They're on the desk," I said as I walked over and opened the plan book for her to see. I began to explain what I was teaching that day, but she cut me off.

"How long is this going to last? I mean, is there an end to this illness that you have? Will you have to keep missing work?" By the agitation in her voice, I knew it was best to walk away, but I couldn't help it.

"Do you think I like being sick?" I retorted. "Do you think I have some control over Lyme disease?" I rolled my eyes and busied myself with some papers. She left without another word.

~

I wanted to walk away, but I could not call it quits. I would not let her force me out. So instead I changed my routine. I stayed in my classroom all day long, except when I had to walk the kids to lunch or a special activity. I avoided the office and the staff room and any other place where I would run into her. I just wanted to do my job and leave.

The new year rolled in along with more intimidation and stress that landed me in the emergency room once again. I noticed a pattern had begun of making progress for a couple of months and then ending up back at the hospital. I was frustrated and angry.

A tingling beehive raging in my head was back and keeping me from sleep. I didn't know how to explain it to anyone, let alone the doctor. It was just there, constantly buzzing, like a vibrating headband. I tried telling my colleagues one day. "You can't sleep, can't think, can't do much of anything because you can't even put thoughts together," I said. The looked at me with blank stares.

At my next appointment, Doc Munshi suggested the next step, a PICC line. Although I respected him as a Lyme-literate specialist and as a doctor, I began to wonder. There had to be other options. I already read up on the PICC line. For many, once you start, you stay on it forever. The PICC line is the beginning of a long road to the end. For many, that end was suicide. I refused that route. I refused to get stuck on any lifelong medication.

~

I had gone from a normal, active, healthy woman to a dying body with a mind that had given up hope. I became a recluse and declined all invitations. Weekend getaways with the girls were refused. My friends didn't understand this disease nor my dietary requirements. Loud music was as irritating as were the looks of pity that people gave me. I wanted my old life back.

Frustrated, I yelled out into the silence of my home, "I WANT MY LIFE BACK!" No one heard. No God listened or else I surely would have been given what I begged for. I gave up.

Then, the phone rang.

"Hi Gail, it's Jennifer, from Cassadaga. Remember me?" she asked. "I want to come over and talk to you about something that may help you. I hear you've been having a hard time with Lyme disease. I think I have something that will help you. I saw a doctor talking about using essential oils for Lyme disease. Is it all right if I come over tomorrow night?"

"I don't know, Jennifer," I said. "I've tried everything. I've been through it all. I'm done. I just don't know what to do anymore." I was on the verge of a breakdown. I was even too tired to talk.

"What do you have to lose?" Jennifer responded cheerfully. "I'll pop in and just give you a few things to try and you never know, just maybe they'll work for you."

She was right. I had nothing to lose. I gave in.

~

The next evening, Jennifer arrived with two other people, and I welcomed them in. I limped over to the dining room table, and we all sat down. They pulled out a binder and handed me papers explaining essential oil protocols for Lyme disease.

Two hours later, after much discussion on the usage of essential oils to help the body heal, they left me with a few bottles of essential oils of oregano, cinnamon, clove, and lavender. I was told to use lemon oil in my water and lavender on my wrists before going to sleep. The girls explained how essential oils worked and told me that this might help with my Lyme symptoms. I didn't believe them, but I didn't want to argue. I was tired.

Every day for a week, I applied the oils to the bottom of my feet, my spine, and then my neck just like they showed me. I used the oils religiously in hopes that they would make a difference.

Then one morning, I woke up and suddenly realized I had slept through the whole night. I sat up in bed and listened. Something was different. It was gone. The buzzing, the beehive in my head, it was gone. The constant in-your-face voice that reminded me I was sick, that I was going to be a victim to Lyme disease forever, was gone. All of it was gone.

There was no grogginess, no brain fog, no blurry thoughts to sort through. I laughed out loud and yelled out in joy even though there was no one in the house to hear me. It made me happy to hear it myself.

I quickly grabbed my phone and called Jen to tell her the good news. I was in tears as I shouted into the phone. She laughed and celebrated with me.

~

As I continued to look for answers, I was led to new books on healing. I came across the work of Dr. Masaru Emoto, a Japanese author, researcher, and doctor of alternative medicine. I read his studies on water consciousness and the effects of prayer, thoughts, and words on water.

Using water crystal images, he demonstrated the power of positive words. I began to wonder how it all related to the water that we drink, the water found all around the earth, and the water in the body. I contemplated the possibility of how we could change the quality of the water we drink simply by praying over it or writing words on the containers that hold the water.

Then another idea came to my mind. My body was nutritionally deprived of essential vitamins and minerals needed for living. If our skin was like a sponge absorbing whatever we put on it, then our bodies could absorb vital minerals by being in the ocean.

Aha! That's why being in the ocean made me feel better, I thought. Then another thought came. *The body is made up of water...what if...* I began to write down my ideas in a notebook.

I researched the health benefits of ocean water and minerals again. Ions were found near oceans and waterfalls. Negative ions in the air around beaches and waterfalls boosted our ability to absorb oxygen, so for someone suffering from air hunger, the ocean was the perfect place to go. Being near the ocean brought greater oxygen to the cells in my body.

Lyme carditis was one of the many symptoms that I faced. It affected the heart. It happened when the bacteria entered the heart tissues and interfered with the electrical signals in the heart. Being near the ocean helped.

I wrote more notes in my binder. Then I began to wonder, *Is this part of the answer to some of the obstacles I've been facing?*

~8~

A Stroke Of Bad Luck

With a new year beginning, I was hoping for breakthroughs, but yawning every few minutes was a sure tale sign of air hunger in me. The added weight on my chest was also a concern that the Lyme had gone into my heart, or so the doctor told me on one visit. Wanting to understand these new phenomena, I took to online research again. I needed more oxygen, and there was something about my red blood cells that they weren't doing their job.

Then a voice in my head said, *You need the ocean.*

I started reaching out to friends and inquiring about cheap beach vacations. I needed to go someplace sunny and near the ocean where I could swim during the mid-winter break from school. Fortunately for me, my college roommate, Kelly, responded and invited me to her home in Key Largo.

She picked me up at the airport, and we chatted nonstop about where our lives have taken us over the few decades since we were in college together. As we came upon the beautiful oceanside community where she lived, I was in awe of the beauty. I gawked at the massive homes adorned with magnificent tropical flowers. I began to imagine what it would be like to live in one of these homes. As a tiny car approached, I asked Kelly what kind of vehicle it was.

"Oh, that's just the neighbors' golf cart" she laughed.

I looked from her back to the tiny car. "That's a Hummer!" I exclaimed.

"Yeah. The golf carts here are a bit fancy aren't they!" Chuckling she went on to explain the line-up of other vehicles as we passed the Yacht Club pool. Looking at the Mercedes, Hummer, and Escalade golf carts that were parked all in a row, I shook my head in disbelief.

"People really live like this?" I laughed. "One of those golf carts probably costs more than my yearly salary as a teacher!" I felt out of place. I tried to imagine what it would have been like to live here as a child. Someone else cleaning the house. No cockroaches skittering between dirty dishes piled high in the sink. And certainly no worry about having clean clothes to wear or dirty old men kissing the children. Hmmph. *Maybe next life*, I thought. For that day, I was just going to pretend I was a celebrity. I put my chin up and raised my hand in a gesture of the princess wave as Kelly and I laughed.

Every day with Kelly was a blessing. Lounging in a hammock with palm trees gently blowing overhead, I looked over at her as she studied for her nursing exams. I closed my eyes and daydreamed about being her neighbor in a tropical paradise. Some of the best moments with Kelly were simply sitting together and laughing with her and her family. Then it occurred to me, laughter had left my life.

~

When I got back from Florida, I was feeling stronger and happier. Then I had a revelation. Whenever I went away to see a friend and was near the ocean, I felt better.

I looked forward to getting back to my classroom and teaching. Then another old friend returned to my life as the phone rang while I sat on my sofa one night.

"Hey, Gail Lynn," he said. "This is Boob! Remember me from the basketball league? Our boys used to play the summer league together."

"Of course, I remember you, Boob," I laughed. "I'm glad you kept the nickname."

"Thanks! Yeah, it kind of stuck with me. Hey, I just heard you've been really sick. I wanted to see how you were doing and if there was anything I could do to help?"

I explained to Boob my last year and a half with Lyme disease and the latest diagnosis of Celiac disease. He offered to come bring dinner over.

"I'm a good cook," he said. "I'll make us some colorful salads and come watch a movie with you Friday night. Unless you feel up to going out dancing," he laughed. I was thrilled at the thought of having company.

For the next six weeks, he was my saving grace. One day he saw the checklist of Lyme symptoms sitting on my table and read through it. He offered his sympathy. He reminded me to take my vitamins and began reading about the essential oils that I was using.

"Let me put some of this on you and see if it will help," he said softly. He grabbed my roller bottles of oregano, cassia, and clove essential oils.

I was hesitant to let anyone touch me because of the pain that radiated up my legs, but he insisted. He was kind and gentle and I was grateful for all his help, but his presence made me miss Bryce. Boob began to hang around a lot, and although I enjoyed his company, I did not have any love interest in him.

~

In school, the vicious cycle of harassment began again. One day at work, I became an easy target of ridicule after posting pictures on social media of my trip to Key Largo. I purposely chose photos that showed me laughing and lounging on the beach. I needed reminders of times that made me laugh. I wanted to surround myself with happy thoughts. My colleagues didn't understand how I really felt. They didn't understand the underlying symptoms that mysteriously appear with Lyme disease.

Throughout each workday, I was seen applying essential oils to my body. I had placed a diffuser in my classroom behind my desk, using wild orange oil to help alleviate stress and thyme oil to support my immune system. I also wore quartz and amber crystals around my neck for their healing properties. My choice of healing modalities was not in line with traditional mainstream healthcare, and it was obvious to everyone at work. I had a different perspective of the medical field, one that no longer aligned with others who saw doctors as godlike sources for answers.

One day the aide in my classroom asked about my treatments. "I sit for spiritual healing in my church," I told her. "I also get Reiki sessions and use alternative healing modalities. Crystals also help; they are minerals from the Earth that have healing properties that support the body. I wear whatever mineral my body needs."

Later that day as I was heading into the staff room for lunch, I opened the door as the aide was saying my name.

"I think Gail has gone a little *woo-woo,*" she told the others.

I stopped walking and stayed right outside the door so she wouldn't see me.

"She has this light thing behind her desk that puts out steam or something and she's always playing strange music. Now she's wearing these crystals around her neck and always wants the lights off. I really think she's losing her mind."

I heard a few laughs as I shut the door. Here I thought the aide was asking about my healing treatments because she was interested. Instead, she just wanted to use it to ridicule me and create the typical staff room drama and gossip. After overhearing a few others talk such nonsense, I began to avoid my colleagues. Going to work each day was getting harder.

A public-school setting was supposed to be a safe place. As teachers, we discipline kids for being bullies, yet the adults get away with it every day in the staff room.

I avoided almost everyone after that. Everyone, that is, except two colleagues, my best friends, Darlene and Deanna. They always came rushing to my side in an instant whenever I had an episode or symptom flare-up at school. Being the center of ridicule became another downward spiral.

~

Many people don't know what Lyme disease is or how it affects people. My doctor, however, reminded me on every occasion that every part of the body is affected and cautioned me at each appointment to avoid stress. Avoiding colleagues, I began to make excuses for their behavior and their jests. At least then it didn't hurt so bad.

I started to eat lunch alone in my classroom and began to write out positive affirmations to make peace with the school's negative environment. I played healing music of Ho'oponopono that I was learning about. Some days, I would lock the door and listen to a guided meditation during my lunch to help erase the fear or sadness.

I also spent my lunchtime conducting more research on alternative healing modalities. I began learning about energy fields around the body and how they can be affected by everything and anything, and then I remembered reading about people who could *read* energy. It made sense and I knew I was one of them. I could detect energy easily. I was an empath, sensitive to feeling the thoughts, feelings, and emotions of others.

Understanding this, even more, I began avoiding people and places that just didn't feel comfortable. I began sensing people's energy as soon as I looked at them or drew near to them, *and* I began to see how everything connected to me as if I were a battery.

Each person, place, or thing had either a positive or negative energy that connected to me. If it was positive energy, I allowed it in my life. If it was negative, I avoided it or eliminated it from my life. Meanwhile, I kept learning and trying to make sense of this ability and its effect on me.

Suddenly I was searching for more answers and not just about Lyme disease, but healing any illness. I could not, would not use any pharmaceutical drugs, nor would I allow any traditional western medicine treatment.

~

During the weeks that I was strong enough to work, the hours between 8:00 am and 3:00 pm were a struggle. Doc Munshi said I didn't allow myself to get strong enough before I jumped back into teaching after each setback. I didn't care. I just wanted my life back, wanted to be normal again. But normal had become different for me. I was learning how to overcome the negative energy of the people in my workplace. I hated that my colleagues were mocking me. I hated that my job was no longer fun. I hated going home alone to a quiet house struggling to find the strength or a reason to keep going.

What's the purpose? I thought.

I hated being different. I hated that I could be reduced to tears by the principal. I hated that she put a poster up on the wall in the cafeteria that said, "Ms. Gail needs help. Walk her students to the stairs." I was reminded of a quote from Robin Williams that I had read after he passed away into the spirit world. He said: "I used to think the worst thing in life was to end up all alone. It's not. The worse thing in life is to end up with people that make you feel all alone."

~

At home, the silence allowed for the reels of film that were in my head to replay over and over. Even the days that

106

my friend Boob stopped over became difficult as his presence made me miss Bryce all the more. All the memories of my ex-fiancé were stuck in my mind like a scratched record that could not move forward to the next note. Our happy memories were covered over by visions of him and another woman. Another woman wearing my helmet, using my bathroom mirror, sleeping on my pillow at his house. Thoughts played like a recording.

You are unworthy, you are alone, you are unloved, you are unlovable, you are unworthy, you are alone, you are unloved, you are unlovable...

My mind was like a projector. The end of the film reel wouldn't stop spinning, the film strip just kept slapping the machine over and over again.

I tried to forget. I tried participating in life, but more often than not, I was just too tired. I spent time with family and friends when I felt strong enough, but even babysitting my own grandchildren was difficult. It tore at my heart every time I had to say no to my son when he asked for help. I couldn't babysit. I was too afraid that I would fail somehow. I couldn't bear that thought.

Then one day, a friend invited me to join her at weekly line dancing lessons. At first, I declined the offer, but after a few weeks of persistence, I agreed. Wednesday evenings soon became a night to look forward to. It fulfilled the latest orders from Doc Munshi to laugh more. It was mid-April of 2015 when I called my friend Jan to invite her to join us as well.

"We're going up to the legion Wednesday night for a line dancing class," I said. "Join us! You can put your cowboy boots to work!"

"Sure!" she laughed. "I've always wanted to try line dancing."

Boob and Darlene ended up going out dancing with us. All night we laughed like silly high school kids as we tried to get the steps down to several dances. Boob ordered us each a glass of wine. We watched him try to do the Cowboy

Cha Cha, determined to impress us. It felt so good to laugh. Then I made my way to our table, exhausted, needing to sit awhile. Boob followed.

"How are you feeling?" he asked. "I was hoping you'd come to check out my new place when we leave. I just moved in this past weekend. I want to show you my new patio that overlooks the lake. It's so pretty."

Boob and I had become good friends. He brought me dinner once a week and got me out of the house when I needed it. He even drove me the three-hours it took to see Dr. Munshi for an appointment once when I didn't want to go alone.

"I don't know," I said. "I'm pretty tired."

"Come on," he persisted. "It's just around the corner. I'll make sure you are home before your curfew." We laughed. "Seriously, come for one glass of wine."

I caved. It was the least I could do after how good he had been to me. It felt good to have someone who cared and expected nothing in return, unlike Bryce.

Boob was proud of his new place that overlooked Chautauqua Lake. *He is a good decorator*, I thought. The water shimmered with the reflection of lights around the shores.

He handed me a full glass of wine and prepared some cheese and crackers.

"Come, sit," he said as he carried a platter of snacks. I joined him on the sofa and grabbed some crackers.

"These are gluten-free?" I asked him before putting one in my mouth.

"Oh, no. I'm sorry. I forgot," he said remorsefully.

"I'm sorry, you know I have Celiac disease. I can't eat them." I tried to cheer him up by making a joke to mimic Doc Munshi's accent. "You'd could die eef you keep eatin da gluten. Is no good for you. You have real bad."

Boob laughed.

"You don't want me to die, do you? Doc would come to hunt you down. He's a good guy. He looks out for me." I smiled.

As we sat on the sofa sipping our wine, Boob looked over at me. "How are your feet after all that dancing?" he asked. "Let me give you a massage. I can put your oils on you and help you to unwind so you sleep good tonight."

Drinking one glass of wine should not have affected me as it did, but my body was sensitive to any drug. I was a lightweight and the few sips of wine already began going to my head. While the thought of a massage was welcoming, I wasn't sure it was the right thing to do.

"I don't know if this is a good idea," I said.

"Come on, let me give you a massage. You know it will help you feel better."

He reached for my purse, handed it to me, and told me to get the essential oils out. Boob grabbed hold of my legs and pulled them up onto his lap. Again, I caved.

He placed a few drops of frankincense oil on my feet and gently rubbed them in.

Leaning back, I closed my eyes and fell into a state of bliss. I reminded him to be gentle. Sighing, I allowed myself to drift off in thought. I imagined feeling better. I imagined what normal and healthy would look like again. Then Bryce popped into my head. I imagined he and I like we used to be.

Then I became aware of Boob's hand as he rubbed further up my leg. Soon his hands had moved up into my inner thigh.

"How does this feel?" he asked.

Feeling uncomfortable, I quickly sat up and reached for my purse. "I'm sorry," I said. "I have to leave."

I stood and headed for the door. "I don't feel good. I have to get home. I'm sorry." I ran out the door. I wanted to get out of there as fast as I could. I needed to clear my head.

What's wrong with you? I mentally berated myself. *You're in love with Bryce. You shouldn't be here with Boob.*

Pulling out of the parking lot, I turned left, toward Bryce's house and began speaking to him in my mind. *What are you doing tonight, Bryce? I miss you.* Within minutes I was driving past his house, wondering if he was sitting in his usual spot on the sofa, with his legs up, falling fast asleep with the television on.

I drove the long lonely road back home with a reel of memories playing in my head. I thought of his proposal and of making love on the beach in the Dominican Republic. I replayed memories of motorcycle rides, camping, wine tours, and horseback riding. We were so passionate about each other. We could be so good together one minute, and then moments later we could part ways.

"WHY...WHY can't we get it to work?" I cried out.

I cried the whole way home. I thought about my life and what a mess it had become. I thought about the job that I had to go to in the morning and wondered how something that I had once worked so hard for had become something that now tormented me. I had more fear and sadness than ever. I was afraid of being shamed again. I feared not being enough, feared being abandoned, feared losing all that mattered to me. The Fear Miser filled my being. Above all, I feared the pain that reared its ugly head and overtook my body without warning.

I felt empty and isolated. I felt unloved and more than anything, tired. Tired of life. As I pulled into my driveway and stared at the vacant house where I had raised my children, I felt more alone than ever. There was no purpose to life, no reason for me to be here.

I reached up to the sun visor, pushed the garage door opener, and watched as the steel wall slowly lifted. Then I pulled forward and pushed the button again and sat there as the wall closed in behind me. Like a prisoner, I was trapped. Inside the garage, it was dark and cold like the confines of a prison cell would be.

I went inside and began pulling off my clothes, leaving a trail as I made my way through the living room, downstairs to my master bedroom. The large master bedroom I once loved had become my dungeon. I didn't bother to turn the lights on. I knew the path well. I slowly climbed into the large king-size bed that engulfed me as I curled up like a baby, hysterically sobbing for that comfort only a parent knows how to offer.

"WHY?" I bellowed.

I held my breath and listened, waited once again for answers, but nothing came. I tried holding in the anger, the fury, the years of agony, but one by one, they all began escaping through pursed lips. I began to pray to God.

God, are you real? Are you here? Why? Why am I so unlovable? Boob doesn't love me. Bryce doesn't love me. Why can't I be loved? Why am I in so much pain? Why does my boss hate me? Why am I ridiculed? Why am I alone? Why does my body hurt so badly? Why do I feel like a worthless old ragdoll tossed out again and again? I can't do this life anymore!

The flood broke as I cried out.

"*TAKE ME!*" I shouted. Grabbing the sheets, I thrashed around on the bed as if wrestling with some entity kicking and screaming with each sob. "TAKE ME HOME! I… DON'T… WANT… TO … LIVE … THIS… LIFE ... ANYMORE!"

I gasped for breaths between words, then finally lay there complete, curled up like a baby, waiting for God to talk to me. Eventually, I fell asleep, wondering what wise words God had for me.

The next morning, I awoke to my alarm ringing. My eyes felt swollen and I was exhausted. So many emotions surfaced as I lay there. I dreaded getting out of bed. I hated the thought of having to go through all the steps of cutting up fruits and vegetables just to have breakfast. I was sick and tired of being sick. I was angry at my boss for not being compassionate. I was angry at her for embarrassing me in front of my students and for mocking my beliefs. My heart began racing.

I do not want to face her today, I thought.

I pushed myself to go to work anyways. Halfway there, my cell phone rang. It was my friend, Jan.

"Hey, friend! How are you this morning?" Her perky greeting was almost more than I could bear. "How was last night at Boob's? Was his place cute?"

What difference does it make if his place was cute, I wanted to say. Materialism is a mask for all that ails you. "I stayed up too late, but I'm fine," I said. "Boob's place was cute."

"I had so much fun!" she continued. "And Boob is a riot!" She continued talking about the songs and dance steps, but I had stopped listening.

A sharp pain jolted like a zap of lightning and radiated down my arm as I pulled into the school parking lot.

"I'm so glad you had a great time," I said half-heartedly. "We'll have to do it again real soon. I'm at work so I have to go."

I turned off the engine and sat in the car for a minute rubbing my arm. First, Bryce crossed my mind. Then I began thinking about the principal and her cleverness whenever she came into my room questioning my ability or worth. I was so tired of this life. I didn't want to go in and face her. I couldn't take being bullied one more day. But again, I forced myself.

Once inside my classroom, I began shuffling through papers on my desk to prepare for the students' arrival when an aide came in.

"Good morning, Gail," she said. "How's your morning going?"

"Not feeling all that well," I said as I sat and looked at her from my desk.

"Yeah, you don't look all that well," she said. "Did you forget you had a meeting this morning?"

"Oh, yes," I sighed. "I forgot. What meeting is it? There are so many meetings. Feels like every day there's something." I shuffled through some papers to find my lesson plan book.

"Do you know where it is?" I asked. My head felt foggy. I couldn't find whatever papers I was looking for.

"I just passed your team in the hallway," she said. "They asked me to tell you to go to the conference room."

I began to gather my things when suddenly I felt even more tired. Exhausted, I sat back down. My arm ached. I mustered up the strength to gather curriculum binders that I needed to bring with me for our team meeting. Then I stood up and handed the morning schedule to the aide.

"If you need any help with students, call the office," I told her wearily. "Yesterday was quite difficult with the full moon. Who knows what today will bring."

As I walked out of the classroom, I suddenly felt lightheaded and dizzy, almost drunk. The left side of my body felt heavy as if it were sagging. I knew I wasn't walking straight. I felt disoriented. I walked down the hallway in a daze until another aide stopped me.

"Oh my, Gail, you don't look good. Are you okay?" She stood in front of me and stared into my eyes.

"I don't know," I said. "I'm tired."

"Where you headed? Do you need help?"

"I have a meeting with my colleagues. I don't know. I... I'm just tired. My head feels funny," I stammered.

"I'm going to walk with you. Maybe you should go sit in the staff room for a bit. Should you even be here? Why didn't you stay at home?"

I explained that I didn't have many sick days left. She led me to the elevator and pushed the button. We took it down to the first-floor staff room where she led me to the sofa. I put my head back and closed my eyes. I wanted to sleep.

"Something's wrong," I said grabbing my arm. "My arm hurts." I pointed to where. "Right here, there's a sharp pain, like I was zapped or something."

"I'm calling the nurse," she stated.

I sensed panic in her voice, but I didn't know why. I was tired and started to drift off to sleep. I heard her voice, but it sounded muffled, and then I heard her again more clearly.

"Where are your oils? Do you want me to call Deanna? Where's Darlene?" Her words all blended like she was babbling.

The next thing I knew, the school nurse was crouched in front of me saying my name. I lifted my head and looked at her. Then Darlene appeared and stood over me looking concerned.

"Look at me, Gail," she said. "What's going on? What happened? I was told to get your bag of essential oils from your classroom and bring them down here."

"I don't know," I sighed. "I'm tired. My arm hurts. I feel foggy."

"When did this start? Do you feel feverish?" Too many questions came all at once.

I mentioned the phone call with Jan on my way to work. "It started… in the car." I struggled to get the words out right. My brain was too tired to think.

I could hear the school nurse asking me questions between Darlene's. "When's your birthday? What is your last name? Open your eyes and look at my fingers. How many fingers do you see?

I thought about the questions. "Mmm…March," I slowly replied. "But … you're talking …too fast."

"What year and date?"

It took me a few minutes to recall the date as if my brain was moving in slow motion, but I finally answered her.

"Gail, we need to get you to a hospital," the nurse said. "I need to call an ambulance. Do you have someone you would like me to call?" She quieted down a bit, but I heard her say to the others, "I think she's having a stroke."

"I'm not…going to a hospital," I sputtered out, looking at Darlene.

I sensed the fear in the nurse's voice as she threw out one question after another. She was too close to my face and it was making me uncomfortable, so I leaned back and closed my eyes again. Somewhere in my mind, I heard her, but I also heard something else. Perhaps they were my own thoughts I was thinking, but it felt as if someone else was talking to me.

I wasn't in pain. Not physically, anyway. I was tired. I just wanted to sleep and not wake up. I thought of Bryce and wished he was there.

"We need to get her to the hospital," the nurse shouted. "I think she's having a stroke."

"No, no hospital!" I shouted back. I opened my eyes and looked up to see Deanna who was now kneeling beside me, watching with concern. She knew my fears about the hospital. She knew my distrust of doctors.

"Let me give her some frankincense," Deanna said to the nurse. "Darlene, get the frankincense out of her bag." Turning and looking at me, she continued.

"Gail, look at me," she said. "I need you to open your mouth and let me put a couple of drops of frankincense under your tongue."

I looked up at the nurse. "Like hell! I'm not going to that place," I said.

"Please," I pleaded with Deanna. "Do not let them take me in an ambulance." The words were loud and clear. I kept repeating myself. "I'm not going to allow this place to get the best of me. I'm not going to let her put me in the hospital again."

I leaned back and opened my mouth. Deanna tipped the bottle of frankincense to get some on her thumb and then put her thumb to the roof of my mouth. I closed my eyes while she held it there until saliva began drooling out the sides. I tried swallowing, but her thumb made it impossible.

"Gail don't bite me," she joked. "I'm trying to help you."

The nurse looked at me in confusion, then turned to Deanna.

"The principal has been harassing her about being sick and her absences," explained Deanna. "We've talked to the teacher's union and the Human Resource director. They both say that they can't do anything because the principal is just doing her job."

The nurse turned to me with a serious look on her face. "Gail, stress kills people every day. This is not worth it. Why are you even here? You need to be home getting healthy."

"I love teaching," I said. "I need to be here. I'm running out of sick days." Tears escaped the corners of my eyes. Feeling defeated, I slumped back and leaned my head against the wall.

"We have to get you to the hospital. It's my job, Gail. I need to make sure you are okay. I need you to stay awake and keep talking to me."

"If Deanna can take me, I'll go," I said firmly. "I'm not leaving this place in an ambulance."

I was afraid that if I fainted, they would allow doctors to start putting pharmaceuticals in me. I thought of my stepmom Sheila who had died in a hospital. I was afraid that incompetent doctors would have a hay-day with me. I needed them to know my beliefs.

"No ambulance, no needles," I stated. "Promise me, Deanna."

The school nurse had a scared look on her face. I think she was afraid I was going to die right there in the staff room. We sat there staring at one another until finally, Deanna agreed to bring me.

"You need a doctor, and you have to let them treat you," Deanna said.

"What do I tell the principal if she comes in?" Darlene asked.

"Tell her I had a family emergency and had to leave to go to the hospital," Deanna said. "She doesn't need to know more than that."

"Please, please don't tell her anything about me," I begged the nurse. "She doesn't need to know my health business. Don't give her a reason to gloat. I'm protected by privacy laws. She has caused enough problems for me."

~

Deanna parked in front of the emergency room entrance then got a wheelchair and pushed me inside. The Fear Miser raged inside me as my mind contemplated what procedures they might try to force on me. The intake nurse began the rounds of questions and I answered best as I could. I told her about the events leading up to being brought into the hospital. I told her of the sharp pain in my arm that occurred on my way to school. I told her of the great amount of stress I felt at work and about the Lyme disease diagnosis.

"I am not a good patient. I'm sorry. I'm afraid. Doctors have misdiagnosed me in the past. It took months to learn I had Lyme disease. I don't trust doctors. I question everything. I don't take pills or medications of any kind."

She just smiled. "Let's get you into a room to be checked out," she said. She pushed me down a corridor into an exam room and began opening packets of what looked like needles.

Nervously, words began coming from my mouth. "I will not take any medications."

She ignored my comment and continued prepping my arm with a cotton swab until I screamed.

"Stop! You are not putting anything into me. What are you doing?"

"We need to get a port in place so that way we can begin to administer medications if needed," stated the nurse, ignoring my pleas.

"No!" I said again. "No, no, no! I do not use any kind of medication. Do not put a needle in me." I pulled my arm away fervently. "I have not had any medications since January 2014, and I will not start now."

The room became suddenly still as everyone stopped and stared at me. "I will not have anything put into me," I said again, only this time in a hushed voice. I lay back and closed my eyes, exhausted, more tears cascading down my cheek.

The nurse put her hand on my arm as if to comfort me. She began to tell me all the reasons why a port was necessary, but I shook my head as she spoke and continued doing so until she pulled her hand back and placed both hands on her hips.

She turned to me and muttered, "Then why come to the hospital if you aren't going to allow us to treat you?"

Her condescending remarks only made me angrier and more ready for a fight.

"Just so you know, I was forced to come here by my employer. The school nurse made me come since I was at work when this began. They made me come here. I didn't want to."

Another nurse chimed in. "If you're having a stroke, which it looks like you are, we have to treat you. Otherwise, there's no sense in you being here. Will you allow us to do an X-ray? And an MRI?"

"No. No X-ray," I answered. "They put out radiation that weakens the immune system. No MRI. Just the bloodwork and tell me the results and then we can go from there." I was steadfast, but after a few more bouts of confrontation with nurses, doctors, and specialists coming in and out of my room, I finally agreed to the MRI.

"At least this will help us to see where the problem is and if there is still a concern we need to address," said one of the doctors. "Based on the symptoms and the admissions report, it sounds like you may have had a Transient Ischemic Attack, so we need to conduct tests to see if there still is a danger of another or a full-blown stroke even."

A short while later, they began prepping me to be transferred to another hospital that was better equipped to handle strokes. What they really meant to say, I think, was that they didn't want to deal with me.

A few hours later we approached the hospital where they specialized in strokes. They whisked me into a room where they began prepping me for more tests. I was not asked nor informed of what was happening. The medical staff just proceeded with tasks. I was fully coherent and watched as they prepped and prepared me and then it hit me that they were about to give me another MRI.

"I had an MRI this morning at the other hospital," I told the nurse. "Why are you going to put me through this again?" I felt like a cross between a guinea pig they wanted to test out and a corpse that they just manipulated. Nothing was discussed with me. The nurse proceeded to get me set for the test and told me to be still, ignoring my question. I was afraid of what they were doing and again felt uncomfortable.

My anxiety level went through the roof until finally, I burst out, "Please stop! I do not do medications and I do not want this done to me. I want to know why you are doing *another* MRI and what you are doing *before* you begin these tests. Please don't put anything into me without my permission." I was angry and raised my voice wanting to be heard.

The nurse rolled her eyes and walked out.

A short while later, a different nurse appeared, although she came in smiling. She reached out her hand to introduce herself and I noticed a butterfly tattoo on her arm with the word "transformation."

Feeling sorry for my outbursts, I tried to be nicer and make small talk with this nurse. Masking my fear, I asked the nurse to tell me about the tattoo on her arm, and she explained its significance to me.

"I'm sorry," I whispered. "I don't mean to be difficult. This is scary. I usually have a friend or someone with me to help me when I'm having medical issues."

I looked away before tears could escape. I didn't like feeling timid or weak. I hated feeling like a coward, but I hated even more not knowing what was happening. I hated that the medical staff never explained anything or asked for my permission to proceed with any treatments.

"I don't believe in medications," I whispered. "Please don't put any pharmaceuticals in my body. I have different beliefs. I am a spiritualist. I use holistic health treatments, and, well, I believe in prayer and meditation to help the body heal. My family should be arriving soon with my essential oils. That is all I use for health care."

I paused before asking, "Do you know anything about essential oils for healing the body?"

The nurse smiled and stated that she also used essential oils. She winked. "I get it," she said. "I would like to do a blood draw though to check to see if your cardiac enzymes are okay." She explained the need for the blood samples and said she would take good care of me and use the smallest needle possible. I finally agreed to allow them to draw a few vials of blood, but that was it.

"Can you at least wait until my family arrives with my essential oils so that I can apply those first?" I asked her.

"Well, what oil will you use and what difference will it make if you use those first?" she asked inquisitively.

"There's an oil called Balance that I use before I have any blood draws," I told her. "I've had a lot of blood taken over the past two years due to Lyme disease, and using Balance essential oil helps the blood flow easier. Otherwise, I have a difficult time. My veins either collapse during the draw or it is very painful. It also helps ease anxiety."

"Oh, I didn't know that," she replied cheerfully. "Well then of course I'll wait until your family gets here. And thank you. That's good to know."

It wasn't long before my daughter-in-law and son arrived with my oils. Alycia asked which oils I wanted first, then began applying them to my feet, legs, and back.

Shortly after, more doctors and nurses filed into the room. "It would be a good idea if you would at least take a baby aspirin," said a doctor. "There's no harm in a baby aspirin, and it will keep your blood thin and prevent you from having any blood clots or another stroke. You had a TIA. That's a mini-stroke. You are lucky it wasn't a full-blown stroke. What happened?" he asked. "When did this all start?"

After explaining my work environment, he nodded.

"Stress can do that. Will you at least take the baby aspirin?"

"I'm sorry, but no. That's why I use essential oils. They're natural remedies. I have not used a pharmaceutical since January 2014."

He shook his head and walked out of the room.

The hospital kept me overnight for observation to monitor my heart. Over the next 48 hours, I continued using frankincense and peppermint essential oil. James and Alycia got my diffuser set up in the room and put in a few drops of frankincense and lavender. Alycia applied lavender on my feet and the back of my neck again before they left that night to help ease the anxiety I was feeling.

The next morning, they ran a few more tests and after the blood draw showed improvements, I was released to go home and told to follow up with my doctor. I would have to see him for a check-up and get a release note stating when I was approved to go back to work. The school district would not allow me to return to teaching until I was seen by my primary care doctor.

~

A few weeks later, I got in to see Doc Munshi. "Because of the stress at your workplace and the TIA, I'm keeping you off work for a while to regain your strength. The stress will continue to cause the Lyme to flare up," he said. "Stress kills people, you know. A stroke is serious business, especially a TIA. It's a warning."

I looked at him, wondering if he was really serious or being funny, but there was nothing playful about his expression.

"You need to do something to manage the stress. What are you doing that makes you happy? Do you have a pet? You need one."

Doc knew I was alone a lot, but I wasn't ready for a pet. I could barely take care of myself.

A few weeks later, I was sitting on my sofa reading some health articles when there was an unexpected knock at the door. I was excited about the idea of company. When I opened the door, I found myself staring at my ex-fiancé. Nervous and confused as to why he was there at my door, coming into my life again, I smiled an awkward smile.

"Um, hi," I said, standing there, shocked.

Bryce laughed. "Hi there, how are you these days?" He grinned from ear to ear as I stood there, wondering if he'd made a joke or if I had missed something.

"Are you going to invite me in?" he asked.

Before I could answer, he stepped forward and placed his arms around me, holding me for a minute in an embrace meant for two people in love.

My body felt the familiarity and responded by hugging him back, though my mind was suspicious.

"Come on in," I said. "Have a seat. What brings you here today?"

"Well," he began, "I heard you had a little trip to the hospital recently and I wondered why you didn't come into my room and say hello. I was there, too." He looked at me again with that same smirk on his face.

Sitting down next to me, we stared at each other. I wasn't quite sure if I heard him correctly. Cocking my head sideways and raising my eyebrows, I waited for him to explain. "What?" I prodded.

"Yes, I was there," he laughed.

"WHAT? Why didn't you call me? You were in the hospital? You were there when I was there? And how do you know that I was in the hospital? And why were *you* there?"

I released a flood of questions, not giving him time to answer one before the next question popped into my head and out through my lips.

"Well, I did call. And you came," he chuckled. "Get it? Telepathically."

I sat staring at him waiting for the next line to say he was joking, but it didn't come.

"I had to have outpatient surgery for a hernia," he continued. "Why were YOU there, and why didn't you call me? If I had known you were going to be there, I would have had you come to visit me. I wanted you there with me."

I thought about those words for a minute and contemplated the significance of them.

"You mean to tell me you had surgery the same day I was in the hospital? AND you wanted ME to be THERE with you? Did you put that thought out?"

We had talked previously about our close connection and being able to read each other's thoughts sometimes or finish a sentence. But this was crazy. Then I remembered my own thoughts that night as I fell asleep before the day of the stroke.

"Bryce, I went to bed that Wednesday night before having a stroke and wished you were with me. I was wishing you and I were together. And then, feeling all alone and hurting all over, I cried out to God and prayed that he would just…you know…take me home. I wanted to die, Bryce. I don't know why you and I have this connection, yet we cannot make it work when we are together. And when we are apart, we want each other. So here we both were in the hospital, both wishing the other was with us." I paused to contemplate what that meant before continuing.

"Bryce, did YOU attract ME to the hospital? Or did I attract YOU to the hospital that Thursday morning?"

He looked at me with tears in his eyes. He reached out and put his arms around me and held me for some time, not talking, just holding me.

When we finally separated, we both wiped the tears away and laughed.

"How long are we going to do this?" he said jokingly.

"Welllll," I drawled it out slowly and playfully. "Do you really feel you needed to end up in the hospital to get me to see you? Couldn't you have just shown up here at my door, just like today? Do you have too much pride to say you're sorry and that you love me?"

"I know how much time you spend at the hospital, so I thought I'd just meet you there," he joked.

We both laughed knowing how much the other hated being in the hospital.

"From now on, can you just call me and plan a date if you want to see me. No more hospital visits. I don't want you in the hospital. I don't want to see you ill. I have never stopped loving you, Bryce. And although I've been hurt by the things you have said and done, I still wish you love and happiness, even if it's not with me. Honestly."

He pulled back his sleeve and looked at his watch then reached for me again. "I have to go. I just wanted to make sure you were okay."

The familiar embrace felt good. Then he pulled back and looked me in the eyes and then slowly leaned in for a kiss. It was soft, gentle, caring. Then he turned and left.

I stood at the door for some time staring off into the distance. My mind became a whirlwind of thoughts, him on one side of the emergency room and me on the other side. It was odd. Life got stranger and stranger by the day.

After he left, I sat for hours wondering about the strange phenomena that seemed to be occurring in my life. I didn't hear from him the next day or the next, but I began reflecting upon many things in my life. I wondered if I had attracted the Lyme disease into my life. The word *attraction* stuck in my head, like the Law of Attraction from the book, *The Secret,* that I had read years ago.

Fascinated at the synchronicity of how events were coming together, I was inspired to pull out some books as I wondered the connection it had to my own life. I wondered if I could truly attract or manifest things into my life. I wondered if I had manifested Bryce and the stroke and the Lyme disease. I wondered if Bryce had manifested me to join him at the hospital and if we had both wanted and created this meeting in the emergency room. So many thoughts ran through my head.

Feeling baffled, I went to my bookshelf and pulled out another cherished book, one with charts about illnesses and their underpinning emotions.

Alphabetically arranged, I turned to letter H and looked up hernias. "Hmm, broken relationships," I whispered. *It makes sense.* Then I turned to the entries with the letter S and read about strokes. Nodding as if agreeing with the author, I spoke quietly aloud. "Yes, I gave up on life. Is it possible? Is it really that simple? Did I create the stroke by my thoughts and the words that I spoke out that night in my fit of anger and despair?"

Right on cue as if answering my question, a soft voice whispered in my ear.

Ask, and you shall receive.

~

Suddenly, everywhere I went, I heard people talking about illness. Everyone had a health issue they were talking about or else they were talking about a family member with an illness. I listened closely to conversations about symptoms and soon came to see how people everywhere were overwhelmed with negative emotions and stress. Worry, sadness, anxiety, anger, fear, resentment, and loneliness were the real illnesses. *Emotions are the cause of ALL illnesses*, I thought.

Digging deeper into metaphysical healing one night, I heard a voice in my head say, *Ho'oponopono*. Then thinking about Shirley from the Women Empowerment class, I tried to remember what she said about this Hawaiian healing practice. Imagining her voice in my head, I pictured her saying the word aloud, "Ho'...o...pono...pono." Shirley broke the word apart allowing us the opportunity to say it ourselves. She went on to explain how she used this Hawaiian practice to offer love and forgiveness to someone who had brought sadness into her life.

I remember Shirley telling us to begin repeating these statements when picturing those who have hurt us:

I'm sorry
Please forgive me
Thank you
I love you.
Ho'oponopono

I closed my eyes and began repeating the words as I thought of Bryce. Then inspired thoughts popped into my head so fast, I could not keep up. And then the man Jesus, who I learned about as a young child, appeared in my mind's eye talking to me.

"Forgive, as you have been forgiven," he said.

I sat on the sofa in dead silence. "What does that have to do with anything?" I spoke aloud as if conversing with the man himself. And then another thought appeared in a vision.

Confess your sins to one another, praying that you may be healed.

The words sang through my head. I looked around my living room as if trying to find the voice that was speaking to me.

My thoughts went to Bryce, and as if I was having a conversation with someone, a voice in my head said to forgive him. Then came the voice again.

Forgive, as you have been forgiven.

I sat there alone in person yet in the company of whoever was speaking in my mind. I did not immediately know who I was conversing with.

Is this what it is like talking with God? I wondered.

Another thought appeared and reminded me of an event in Lily Dale in 2014 with the author, Neale Donald Walsch. Perhaps this was how he had come up with his book, *Conversations With God.* I remembered something Neale said that day when he told a story to illustrate the effects of sorrow. He shared how he had an imaginary conversation with a person and asked the individual, "What hurts you so much that you have to hurt others?" In further dialogue, he brought to my awareness that hurting people hurt others. Then I thought about how this could relate to Bryce and me.

I sat for a few minutes pondering what words to say and then began talking out loud. "Bryce, I'm sorry," I said. "I love you. Whatever harm I caused you, I'm sorry. Please forgive me." I stuck to repeating these words whenever he came to my mind over the next few weeks, and a month later, he showed up at my door again.

We talked for several hours when suddenly the thought in my head got louder and louder.

Tell him you're sorry.

Confused, I looked around as if the voice was coming from outside of me, somewhere in the house. Then I looked at Bryce sitting next to me and heard it again.

"Bryce," I finally said. "I want to tell you something. I need to tell you something. And I want you to listen carefully because it's important."

He turned serious at the sound of my voice. "What is it?" he asked. "Is something wrong?"

"Do you remember the Fourth of July two years ago? When I ran into you at the bar in Dunkirk. You were with someone–"

"We don't need to talk about that," he cut me off. "It was a long time ago."

"Bryce, I need to talk about it. I need to say I'm sorry. I said some harsh words to you and looking back, I feel bad. Seeing you with another woman hurt me, and I

127

wanted to hurt you back. But I know now that I was wrong. And I'm sorry. I love you. I don't want to hurt you. Will you forgive me?" Tears ran down my face.

"We don't need to talk about the past," he insisted, his eyes welling up.

"Bryce, I'm sorry. Will you forgive me?" I asked again.

He reached over and put his arms around me, drew me in for a warm embrace. "Yes. Yes, I forgive you," he whispered. "But let's just look forward. Let's think about where we can go from here." He pulled back and looked into my eyes. Brushing a tear away, he stared into my eyes. "I want to stay here with you tonight. Can I stay?"

"Yes. You can stay," I replied. I looked at the clock and saw the time. "It's almost midnight," I said. "I'm tired. I want to fall asleep in your arms. Are you ready to go to bed?"

My heart was at ease. I truly meant what I said to Bryce. We went to sleep that night wrapped up in each other's arms tighter than we had ever before.

In the next few months, we were inseparable. Either I spent the night at his house, or he was at my house. Part of me thought that our close encounter with death gave us this opportunity to make our relationship right. A few months passed. Things were going well. I was making progress with my healing and the Lyme disease and the summer was stress-free. In September, I was back to teaching again, and along with working came the stress again.

Days were stressful, but nights still consisted of time with Bryce cooking dinner side by side and sharing our life. We held hands everywhere whether we were sitting on the sofa or walking in a store. We fell asleep in each other's arms and awoke the next morning the same way, our bodies intertwined whenever they could. Our love, it seemed, kept growing deeper and deeper. Our love and evenings of joy together kept the stress from taking over, although, after a while, little symptoms began to appear. Frequent yawning from a lack of oxygen was a sure tale sign that stress was invading again and the cells in my body were oxygen-deprived.

Frustrations began arising next as my special diet became a nuisance and began to fall through the cracks whenever I was at his house. He *forgot* that I needed to eat gluten-free, and he made meals that my body couldn't tolerate. He became frustrated, and I became angry. I tried ignoring the symptoms and pretending I was fine, but symptoms only worsened. Between stress at school and stress from worrying that Bryce would get upset with me, I began having heart palpitations

The Lyme disease had a mind of its own. The on and off symptoms were mirroring my relationship with Bryce. I had the symptoms under control, but as soon as I began putting Bryce before my own needs, just like when I put my job before my own needs, symptoms began to reappear.

We broke up again before the year came to an end. Christmas was difficult and 2016 began with greater heart problem issues. As I tried to ignore the pressure each day, my life was going through highs and lows of all kinds. I forgot about Bryce by dating another man. I pretended I was feeling good when inside I felt like everything was wrong. Heart palpitations only added to the problem at work as I tried to manage two flights of stairs throughout the day which became another battle. After another month of pushing myself to the limits, a sick day had me at a doctor's office for blood work that led to a diagnosis of chronic anemia and yet another period of time off from work.

My body was struggling to make red blood cells, and the doctor said I could die if I didn't get to the hospital for a blood transfusion right away. I was scheduled immediately and told to have someone drive me in.

Frightened with the latest bit of information, the doctor took me off work for the remainder of the school year to get my iron and red blood cells healthy again. Advised to begin getting shots to help build my immune system, again I declined, preferring to help my body only through holistic means. Fresh beets, molasses, and Vitamin B Complex with Folic Acid were my newest treatment along with doing what I could to reduce worry and stress, both taxing on the production of red blood cells.

Referring to holistic research, I read in a medical research paper that anemia is related to stress and feeling a lack of joy as well as fearing something in life, or not feeling good enough.

Well, I thought, *avoiding stress and finding something to be joyful about would help me stay out of the hospital.*

Needing to be around other people, I decided to go to Lily Dale for a walk. I ran into an old friend at the boathouse and we talked about life and things that would make us happy. "I WANT A HOUSE RIGHT HERE ON THE LAKE!" I stated adamantly.

Two weeks later, I heard of a house for sale in Lily Dale that had something I had always wanted, a backyard on the lake. I immediately drove to the house and spoke with the owner. Within a few weeks, the house was mine. Now I had two houses to take care of.

Taking the summer to heal was just what I needed, although healing wasn't happening fast enough. When September rolled around, I wasn't sure if I had it in me to return to teaching. I had some good, but more often than not, life was lonely and tiresome. Working through symptoms day after day, I was fed up. I arranged for a meeting with the school union to discuss an early retirement.

Frustrated with yet another setback, I broke down and drove to the local New York State Disability Office. Walking in the door, I immediately felt it wasn't the right thing to do. A voice in my head kept repeating, *Quitter, quitter.* So instead of sitting and talking with the administrator, I took the papers with me and said I would return them the next day. But when I got home, I threw the papers in the garbage. "I'm NOT a quitter!" I yelled out.

I made a deal to give it one last try. I met with the teacher's union again and said I would attempt to return to school with the promise that the principal would stay away from me. Explaining how every interaction with her caused great stress, I pointed out the pattern of being brought to the hospital after each meeting with her.

As it was, a past school board member was the grandfather of one of my students. He offered to volunteer in my classroom a few times a week. After that, things got better and better each month. The principal was no longer coming into my room to harass me and I was able to make greater progress with my health. I liked that man. He became my protector.

Fall turned to winter and then a new year began. I felt the urge to get back to my writing and so the next day I bought a new journal. It was the start of a new year and it deserved a new journal. On the front page, I wrote, "2017: The Year of Manifesting." And then, I decided to put our family house up for sale. *I need a new start*, I thought. I decided to move into my house in Lily Dale full time. Making that decision was scary. I questioned whether I was ready to give up the home where I raised my children, the place where family dinners and holidays came to be so important.

Surprisingly, Bryce showed up again. It was two days before Valentine's Day. As our usual pattern went, I let him in, we talked, we made up, we began dating again. This time, I was a little stronger. I was more secure with myself. There was no mention of the time on Valentine's Day when he had proposed years back. It was as if it never happened.

One day I heard that a favorite author of mine, Ester Hicks, was coming to the area, and I called my friend Denise to see if she wanted to go with me to the conference.

"Let's do it!" Denise said excitedly. "I'll ask my fiancé if he wants to join us. He listens to Ester all the time."

"Okay," I said. "I'll ask Bryce if he wants to go. He hasn't really shown an interest, but it would be nice if he came along and heard this."

I called Bryce and just as I figured, he didn't want to go. He wanted to go four-wheeling in Virginia instead. After a short conversation about trying to persuade him to join us in attending the event, I finally gave up.

"I figured we'd be going four-wheeling," he grumbled.

"Honey, we can go four-wheeling anytime, Ester Hicks only comes once a year. I'll even pay for our tickets," I said excitedly.

"No," he repeated. "I'm going four-wheeling. Do what you want."

"You can't take one day and do something with me that I enjoy?" I waited, hoping he would change his mind.

Dead silence.

"I don't want to go to some stupid conference. It's my day off." I hung up the phone with him and sat in silence.

No more was said about the subject, but throughout the week my heart became heavy. A voice in my head that was not quite audible, kept saying, *Let go.*

For years, I had tried to break the tie between Bryce and me, yet we always ended up back together. *Why can't we break this bond that we have? What is this tie that keeps us hooked together?* I asked myself.

One day as I was leaving school, my friend Darlene stopped me.

"Is Bryce planning anything for your birthday coming up? It's the big 5-0. You need to have a big party!" She stood staring at me with bright and eager eyes. I wanted to be excited, but I didn't know how to answer her.

"I don't know," I said. "I'm not sure how much longer Bryce and I will be together. I don't think he's even thinking about my birthday. You know I'm always walking on eggshells with him. Besides, I haven't been feeling very well."

"Come on," she persisted. "It's the BIG 5-0! We need to celebrate. If Bryce doesn't want to plan something for you, and if your kids aren't planning anything, then I will. I'll figure it out."

A few days later, I got a call from my friend Denise.

"Hey, dolly," she said playfully. "I got a call from Darlene. She said she's throwing you a party! I can't wait! What does the birthday girl want?"

"I don't want a party," I let out. "I want to get away from here, away from work, and the memories of Bryce, and this sickness and all of it."

"What happened? Are you okay?"

I explained how symptoms had returned and began to slow me down. "I'm extremely exhausted all of the time, and the heart palpitations are getting worse again. It scares me. When I'm at work, I crawl under my desk and sleep during my lunchtime. Walking up and down the stairs gets me winded. I'm not sleeping at night, and Bryce and I won't last much longer."

"I'm sorry, Gail," she said. "Why don't you book a trip to Hawaii and go stay with my sisters over spring break? Hawaii would do you good."

I laughed. "Me? In Hawaii? That's only for lovers and honeymooners," I sighed.

"Just think about it," she insisted. "You know, I've mentioned this to Wendy once before, and she and Laurie would love to have you come to visit. Why not treat yourself to Hawaii for your birthday? The flights are pretty reasonable right now."

The thought of me going to Hawaii by myself sounded ridiculous and far-fetched. But something came over me as if someone else was in control. "Fine. I'll go," I pouted as if someone just had to twist my arm into doing something difficult. Over the next few days, I wasn't sure if I was excited or worried.

When the weekend arrived, Bryce came over for dinner. Sipping my wine, I asked him if he had made any plans for my birthday.

"Why should I make plans? That's your kids' job."

"I didn't say you had to make plans Bryce. Darlene asked me if you were doing anything. She wants to plan a party."

"Well tell her to go ahead then."

"Okay, I will." Then taking a bigger gulp, I went on. "Just so you know, I made a plan to go to Hawaii to visit Denise's sisters over my Spring Break. I'll be there for ten days."

"WHAT?" Bryce snapped his head back around to look at me. "What do you mean you're going to Hawaii? What about me? You're going without me?"

"Yes, I need some quiet time to relax and forget about everything for a while. Besides, you–"

"You know what," he interrupted. "I'm done. You want to go do things on your own, then go." He picked up his keys and walked out while I sat there dumbfounded.

I looked around my living room as if an angel would appear. I closed my eyes, placed my hands over my heart, and prayed.

Dear God, being in this relationship with Bryce keeps hurting us. Why do we keep getting back together just to continue the heartache? I'm sorry for whatever I have done in the past that hurt him. I'm sorry if our previous life ended in heartache for him or me, but I can't do this anymore. And every time we try to part ways, we fight our way out hurting each other more. Can't we just simply go our own ways easily, without pain and suffering? I don't want to fight with Bryce. I wish only happiness for him. I wish him love. It's not me that makes him happy, so fine, let it be with someone else. Just let it be over gently. Don't let it hurt.

I sat there allowing the tears to fall, allowing myself to feel the sadness that comes with goodbye. Closing my eyes, I brought Bryce to my mind. I saw him sitting on his sofa, feet up, and his eyes closed sleeping to the sounds of the television. In my mind, I spoke to him.

I love you, Bryce. I always will. I want the best for you, but it seems like that isn't me. I don't know how to make you happy and myself happy too. I asked God to help you find love and happiness. You'll find it, someday. Don't go far.

Climbing into bed that night, the thoughts continued. I pulled out my journal and wrote:

> Dear God, Source, Creator, Intelligence ... I don't understand my life. Who the hell are you? Did I manifest this illness? Can you take away this pain? What is this tie between Bryce and me? Please take away the karma that binds us together. Please heal and mend whatever that is between us. It hurts too much. I'm sorry Bryce for whatever harm I have caused you. I am sorry if my family has hurt you or your family. Please forgive me. Thank you. I love you.
>
> Oh Universe, please let this end in a gentle way without friction or more pain in my soul. We have passed the time that we could be together in this lifetime. Please heal that relationship and allow me to move on. Please help him to move on. I can't go on like this anymore.

~

Between my birthday on March 26 and leaving for Hawaii in mid-April, I had to stay healthy enough to travel. The stressors were coming on faster and stronger. Each morning, I pushed myself to be positive about my day at school. When I came home, I had to pack up my belongings from the last twenty years. My house sold and the new owners would be moving in on the very day that I left for Hawaii.

Saying goodbye to our home was harder than I thought it would be. Trying to decide what to pack, what to sell, what to give away, what to store became overwhelming. My children were busy with their lives and wanted no part of sorting through the years of our memories. I couldn't blame them. My heart was heavy as I walked room to room trying to figure out what to do with all the stuff accumulated over the twenty years.

Days away from having to be out of my house and boarding a plane for Hawaii, I didn't have it in me to go through another box, another closet, or another storage room full of memories of my years of marriage and raising my children.

I called an old pastor friend of mine and told him to come and pack up everything that was left and take it to Goodwill or use it for the church. I couldn't face another loss. I stayed in my kitchen and packed up what was left there as he loaded and took away two trailers worth of my life. The following day I packed a suitcase for Hawaii and made my final walk through the home.

What happened to my life? I asked God, but there was no response. I drove to Denise's house and stayed with her for the night. I fell asleep on her sofa with tears slipping out of the corners of my eyes. Spring break was just what I needed. I was going to Hawaii. Happy birthday to me.

The long flight was worrisome and contemplative. When I finally arrived in Hawaii, Wendy and Laurie, Denise's sisters, greeted me with the traditional Hawaiian lei. I forgot all my cares and was immediately in awe of the surroundings.

"Aloha, Gail Lynn!" said Wendy. "It is so good to have you here in Hawaii!"

I felt like a little girl being handed the best Christmas present ever. I looked around and took in all the sights, all the beauty. I immediately felt at peace, felt loved, felt accepted. It felt like home.

"We know you eat healthy," Laurie laughed. "Instead of trying to guess at what you needed, we're going to stop and let you pick things out at our little store, the Island Natch. Maybe you can teach us a thing or two about eating healthier."

Over the next week, they took me on long drives around the island to see the coastlines covered with tropical flowers. They took me to see beautiful waterfalls, and the warm ponds where I soaked in sulfur infused ocean water from the lava of Pelé, the volcanic goddess. Once, while floating in the middle of the warm pond, I thought of Dr. Emoto's work and closed my eyes and asked the water to heal me.

I began to have visions of childhood experiences long forgotten. Watching little children running barefoot through the grass triggered more early childhood memories. In an instant, I felt a great loss for the childhood I had missed out on. Tears were released from the corners of my eyes and joined the salty sea.

Each morning upon waking, Laurie would hand me a cup of coffee and tell me to come and sit with her out on the lanai. Listening to the birds as the morning sun rose, she opened a book to read the daily inspiration. I felt pampered and taken care of as both Wendy and Laurie saw to it that my spirit was nourished each day.

"Today we are going to see a woman who has been training with a shaman," Laurie said one morning. "The indigenous Hawaiians know secrets to healing. I thought you might like talking with her."

I smiled. By night's end, I wanted to know more about shamanic practices and have a better understanding of how sickness enters the body, so Wendy found yet another shaman to learn from.

On another day, we went to a sound healing event with a practitioner who bathed us in melodies from Tibetan singing bowls. Learning about vibrations and healing from music, I began to research these as healing modalities and the science behind them.

The week went by in a flash. Before I knew it, it was time to go back to New York. Of course, I wasn't ready to leave. With a heavy heart, I told Wendy that I felt like I was just beginning to learn, and there was so much more to uncover.

"Gail Lynn, you have the whole summer ahead of you," she said. "Come back then and stay as long as you want. Stay the whole summer if you can. Let Hawaii heal you."

The return home was long, but it gave me time to contemplate the week. I was excited about the life in Hawaii that I had just experienced, and I was excited to learn more about the ways of the shaman and more about Huna and Ho'oponopono and Aloha.

~

When I finally arrived home that afternoon, I felt different. I sat in my car for a few minutes in front of my house contemplating what I left and what I was returning to. Hawaii captured my heart and I knew I had to go back. Taking a deep breath, I turned to face the old life I had left behind.

Opening the door to my enclosed porch, I stepped inside noticing a large black garbage bag sitting smack center in front of the main door. Surprised, I set my suitcases down and wondered who had left me a gift. Peering inside, I saw the ivory crocheted dress that Bryce had gifted me to wear for his last proposal. It lay crumpled in a heap at the bottom of the bag. My body froze and my heart began to race. I pulled out the dress and saw a few books, a red crystal heart he had given me, my brush that was in his bathroom, and our plant.

I was beside myself. The ecstatic happiness that I brought back with me from Hawaii was suddenly gone. I set everything back in the bag and took my suitcases inside, leaving the garbage bag on the porch. Anger swept over me.

I went back to the porch, grabbed the garbage bag, and headed to my car. I drove the thirty-five minutes to his house. His truck wasn't in the driveway. I left the bag and the plant, now with its broken leaves, on his doorstep, then drove to the grocery store to pick up some food and a new plant for a new start.

By the time I got back home, I was aghast. The large black garbage bag and plant were *back* on my porch. I was furious. I didn't even bother to go inside. I picked up the plant and the bag and sped back to his house.

Pulling into his driveway, Bryce stood there staring at me with a smirk on his face. I got out of the car with the bag and plant in hand and marched right up to him.

"Bryce, why are you doing this? We are done!" I exclaimed. "I do not want any connection to remain between us. I won't wear the dress ever again so give it to your sister or your next girlfriend. I do not want anything in my house related to you or our past relationship. As much as I have loved you, we need to stop this. I just got back from Hawaii, and I want to cut all ties from our past. If you don't want these things, then throw them away." I stared at him and waited for him to take them.

He stood there staring at me. Then he slowly reached out and took the items from my hand. I was about to turn and walk away when he reached out and grabbed my hand.

"You know we have a connection," he said. "We will always have a connection." He pulled me into an embrace and gazed into my eyes then leaned in and planted a kiss on my lips. It felt warm, familiar. I was under his spell once again as our bodies met. I tried to pull back, but he only drew me in tighter, parting my lips with his tongue. Pressed against him, I could feel the pounding of our heartbeats. I began to kiss him back.

Releasing me ever so slightly, he breathed into my ear. "I love you." We stood there embracing for another moment as our hearts beat wildly. "Come inside and have a glass of wine with me. Let's talk." His eyes glistened as the afternoon sun caught what appeared to be a tear in his eyes.

My head yelled don't do it, but my heart caved. I went inside.

He poured two glasses of wine then handed me one. "Cheers," he said, half smiling. We both took a big sip.

"Bryce, what do you want in life? What do you want from me? What do you want in a relationship? I cannot keep having my heart broke every time you walk away from our relationship." We sat in the silence just looking into one another's eyes. Then an idea came over me.

I grabbed the yellow sticky notes that were sitting on the counter and handed one to him. "Think about what you want in life," I said. "Think about life and where you want to be a year from now or five years." I turned away so he couldn't see as I drew a picture of my own. I drew a house, a yard, a garden, a large driveway with many cars, a retreat center, and two people, a couple, on the deck talking with others. I covered it up and handed him the pencil for him to draw his own.

When he was finished drawing his picture, he slid it over to me. "I want a suitcase filled with a million dollars," he said.

I showed him my picture. "Bryce, nothing in your drawing has anything to do with us. That's why it doesn't work. What's important to you is money, material things. What's important to me is time with people I care about, having a retreat center someday, teaching, sharing all this life with you." I slid my drawing over for him to see. At that moment, I knew we were in different places and wanted different things in life.

He pushed aside the sticky notes and pulled me down off the chair. He led me through the kitchen, past the living room, and up the stairs to his bedroom. Standing at his bedside, his hands reached out and began lifting my shirt up and over my head. I didn't resist. Leaning in, our lips met, soft and slow at first, until passion arose, and his warm tongue began descending my neck to my breasts. Both of our hands were now frantically undressing each other. As he picked me up and gently placed me upon his bed, I moaned, longing for that connection that our bodies understood.

We spent the night loving each other unconditionally. Our arms and legs intertwined, hot and sweaty from the ecstasy we experienced once again. We fell asleep holding each other tight.

The words of William Law rang in my heart, "Love has no errors, for all errors are the want for love."

~

The next morning was a typical morning with Bryce. We showered together, taking care to wash our most intricate parts. He put shampoo in the palm of his hand, rubbed them together, and massaged my head.

"I know you like this," he smiled. I closed my eyes and savored the moment. Then he gently pulled me into the stream of water to rinse my hair. When we both finished washing the other, he gently kissed me and said he was going to make coffee.

I finished up, dried my hair, and got dressed. He returned with a cup of coffee. "Breakfast will be ready shortly," he said.

I gathered my things and went downstairs. The smell of bacon greeted me just as he set our plates down. "Smells yummy," I smiled. "I'm starving. Thank you."

He was suddenly sullen as he sat down. We both knew what was coming and couldn't ignore it any longer.

"We had a nice night together," I tried. "But now what? It never seems like I'm enough or that you are willing to stick it out with me. You need to figure out for yourself what you want." He sat there in silence, eating his eggs and playing with the bacon strips on his plate.

We finished eating and washed up the dishes. "I have to go home now," I continued. "I have suitcases to unpack and I'm meeting Denise later for dinner." I grabbed my coat and went to the door then turned to look at him. It was hard to stand there. We're never taught how to say goodbye to someone we love.

"Well, I guess I better go," I said. He did not attempt to stop me, so I walked right out the door, got in my car, and drove home.

The following week, school was back in session. I was still on a high and thinking a lot about the healing the island offered me. I wanted to go back for more. As the days passed, I began to read more about healing through alternative modalities and shamans and I journaled how it related to my experience in Hawaii. I started with my journal entries from many years ago and made note of major events that had occurred over my life.

Suddenly my phone went off with an alert. It was Bryce's birthday. Contemplating what to do about it, I thought about him being alone for his birthday and my heart felt sad. I gave him a call.

"HEY! Happy birthday!" I said. "Do you have plans tonight?"

"Not yet. I was going to call my sister to see if they wanted to go grab something, but I'd rather see you if you're free."

I picked him up and asked him what he felt like eating for his special day. He chose to eat at Taco Hut. He was quieter than usual. We were cordial with each other, made small talk, but nothing more. He wasn't himself and I felt bad. When we got back to his house, he invited me in.

"I don't think that's a good idea. I plan to head back to Hawaii after the school year is over in June." He turned his head away just as his eyes began to glisten.

"You know I love you, Bryce. I will *always* love you, and I'll always be there if you need me."

"I love you, too." He reached over and hugged me, then opened the door and got out. Walking to his door, I waited for him to turn around and wave. I pulled out of his driveway and waved back. I knew it would be a long time before I would see him again.

~

April turned to May and my longing for Hawaii grew. I was elated thinking back to September when I was almost ready to throw in the towel. It was the longest period of time I had gone without a setback. Almost a whole year with no hospital or doctor visit.

I dug out all my books on healing and laid them out on the floor and sat in the middle of them. Then I pulled out more books from metaphysical authors that I had studied and added them to my pool of books. I began to sense that the information from all these authors put together would indeed make a difference in my life, would indeed lead me to my next lesson or my next teacher.

I suddenly remembered my story I had started writing in 2014, after teaching a class in Lily Dale called, *Take Back Your Life*. I found it and rifled through it, a collection of poems and short stories from over the years.

I crossed off the title and wrote in its place, *The Spiritual Truth of Healing: My Journey Back to Health*. I searched my laptop for files with the most current date and began working diligently over the next few days to read, edit, and outline chapters. I felt a new determination. I was going to take back my life *and* I was going to go on a health journey this summer in Hawaii. I was going to get whatever I needed to heal once and for all. Complete wellness would be mine. No more doctors, no more pills. I was even open to the idea of not having to use the essential oils. I wanted perfect health again!

I began writing every day. I knew something was leading me, I felt it. I listened to Wayne Dyer's podcasts each day on my way to work, and his words reinforced my decision to go back to Hawaii as he told stories about living in Maui and the healing he experienced there.

"One day, Wayne," I spoke aloud. "One day I am going to carry that torch of love, hope, and inspiration just like you did."

As if on cue, I came across an advertisement for the Hay House Writer's Workshop 2017 in Maui. When you finally decide to follow your heart, your bliss, and your desire to seek the truth, then you will begin to notice even more patterns, signs, and omens left for you by the angels, by the Universe, and by the great All-Knowing. As I received little nuggets of information, I begin laying them down together like a puzzle that the universe had given me one piece at a time.

That one week in Hawaii had me hooked. I was going back to find greater healing, to find the answer as to why I had this illness. I was going to be my own knight in shining armor, my own hero! I was going to find out how to overcome it once and for all.

I spoke to the island in my heart. *Oh Hawaii, can you bring me healing? Can you make me whole again? What gifts do you have to offer me?*

I read more about the writer's workshop and instantly booked a reservation. Then I searched for a flight to Maui and booked that, too. It felt hasty, but I knew Hawaii had the answers to my healing.

~9~

Follow Your Heart

Consumed with the thought of making my body stronger and ridding the Lyme disease once and for all, I went from bookstore to bookstore buying six, seven, even eight books at a time. I bought books on food, energy healing, shamans, and past life memories. Finding a book that addressed healing through writing, I was more excited than ever. It was confirmation from the Universe that I was supposed to go to Maui to the Hay House Writer's Workshop.

I read the work of Catherine Jones, who discussed the idea that stories about our past, told through focused journal writing, can bring healing and empowerment. I dug into that idea and began to implement personal journaling each night more intentionally.

I also began incorporating some writing ideas with my third-grade students, using the writing process to help them solve problems in their daily life. Making this connection between writing and releasing emotions for my students began to curb their disruptive behaviors that occurred each day. Writing out their feelings was a new coping strategy, and better yet, writing was no longer a chore for these eight-year-olds. Together we were creating solutions to their problems and they were writing for a good reason.

We were now in our last few weeks of the school year and students were suddenly eager to write. A dozen of my children walked into the classroom one morning and were excited to have me read their stories. I was pleased with this newfound love of learning that many of them had found, this love for writing.

"You are becoming authors!" I praised them.

Their stories contained their thoughts, feelings, and worries about so much, from a pet dying, to parents in jail, and even about me heading to Hawaii to get my health back. One student waited until the end of the day to set her story on my desk before leaving school one afternoon. In her story, she shared her sadness about the school year ending and saying goodbye to me. In a few short paragraphs, she transformed that sadness into hope, not only for a beautiful summer but also for my healing as her teacher. The compassion that came out in her story touched my heart to the core.

Our classroom became a writer's workshop for the last month of school where we all expressed our feelings of excitement for the summer vacation coming but also our sadness for the goodbye that was coming as well. Like me, they wrote about their fears of what lay ahead.

As the end of the school year drew nearer, I began to tell my students about my upcoming trip to Hawaii to heal the sickness I had for so long. They were happy for me. As I shared with them my fears, they too opened up more about their concerns. I shared with them how writing had helped me and how I was going to go to a conference to learn how writing helps us feel better. I was excited to share with them pieces of my own writing. Leaving school each day after dismissal, I now had a skip in my step.

"Must be the principal is finally leaving you alone," one colleague laughed as she watched me close my door for the day.

"Well, yes," I said with a grin. "I stay in my classroom all day. I only leave to walk students to lunch or their special class. I have my aide get my mail from the office, so I don't have to go in there either. I have avoided running into her at all costs AND it has paid off."

Two weeks before leaving for my summer healing journey to Hawaii, I couldn't help but share my excitement with my colleagues.

"That's not why I'm so happy though," I said. "I'm leaving for Hawaii soon and will be gone for the whole summer! I'm using some alternative health modalities to finally get over this Lyme disease, the Celiac disease, and I'm going to get my life back!" I was ecstatic at the idea of being healthy and whole again, of living a normal life again.

"Really?" they asked. "When do you leave? You'll be gone the *whole* summer? What about trainings?" Questions fired out at me without a single show of support. I was shocked that not one person was happy that I was going away to get better.

The news spread quickly. The following day the principal showed up at my door just as I was gathering my things to leave for the day.

"I hear you're going away for the summer," she began. "What are you going to do about the summer workshops?" She stood glaring at me with her arms crossed as if waiting for a response.

Like a robot in monotone, I returned to her my sentiments. "Talk to the teacher's union if you have a question about my summer vacation."

I busied myself packing up my things to leave. I didn't want to get caught in a conversation alone with her as she so often had done before. The conversations never ended well.

"Well, we'll see what HR has to say," she scoffed before turning and walking away.

I shut off the light and closed my door then walked away in the opposite direction. I didn't want to give her another opportunity to say anything to provoke me or cause any undue stress. I had made it this far, and I wasn't about to let her agitate me or send me back to the hospital. I would not let her get under my skin.

~

As old habits die hard, I began to worry over what her next action would be. I expected her to try to make that last week hell for me. She couldn't stand it that I was happy, but I was determined to stay strong. I was adamant that I wasn't going to let her get in the way of me getting my life back. I had come to the conclusion that if I didn't have my health, my job would be meaningless anyway. You have no life if you don't have your health. My career, my pension, all of it would be worthless if I had to keep running back to the hospital every three months.

I will not let her bully me anymore, I thought.

The next day, however, I reverted to my old ways. I was anxious, terrified actually, that I would run into the principal. And worse yet, I was afraid stress was going to cause another setback in symptoms and prevent me from going on my trip. I was afraid I was going to end up back in the hospital. Throughout the day, I took extra care to remind myself to stay calm.

While the students were in lunch, I sat in my classroom, used my mala beads, and stated affirmations with meditation music instead of eating. When lunch was over, I went to pick the students up from the cafeteria. That's when the assistant principal came up to me and began whispering under her breath.

"Gail," she said quietly, looking around to see if anyone was watching us. "You need to contact the Equal

148

Employment Opportunity Commission and file a complaint. The principal is not going to stop bullying you unless you do something. You are a weak victim to her." She lowered her voice even more. "She makes comments to me all the time about you being a *witch*, she makes fun of you and the whole Lily Dale community. She even said you put a spell on her. She has told me to go to your classroom multiple times a day to watch you and question you. She wants me to push your buttons. Heck, she's the one who told me to do a surprise evaluation on you the last time you came back from the hospital. She knew you would get upset."

I stood there staring at her trying to comprehend what she just said to me. Rethinking her words in my head, I asked myself if she really used the word *witch*. I needed to know if she was serious. "Did you say the principal called me a witch? Like a *real* witch? Or was she just saying I act witchy? What do you mean?" I laughed trying to make light of the situation.

"Gail," she paused, making sure I was looking at her. "Seriously, she is bullying you because she is afraid of you. She thinks you put a spell on her. She really thinks you are a witch, and she blames you for her falling off a ladder. Don't you see? You have a case of discrimination here. Not only because you have been sick and out on disability with Lyme disease but also because of your religious beliefs. She's spreading rumors about you."

My head was spinning. I didn't know what to think. The principal actually believed that I was a witch. The look on my face must have said it all because the assistant principal laughed again.

"I don't understand any of this," I said. "I would never hurt anybody, nor is there such a thing as witches." I stood there shaking my head in disbelief at the whole conversation.

"Listen," she looked around and leaned in closer again. "You know those videos all the teachers have to watch every year at the beginning of the school year? Watch them again. One of them is about bullying in the workplace. Have your colleagues help you document all the interactions you've had with her. You have a case. There are laws against what she is doing, and your union should be protecting you. I can't say more. She's probably watching us on the cameras here in the hallway. If she is, she's going to question me. If she asks, I'll say I was talking to you about your lesson plans. Call the office of the EEOC."

"What is the EEOC?" I asked, more confused.

"Look it up." She turned and started to walk away then paused and looked back. "One more thing, if you don't believe me that the principal called you a witch, then call your ex-colleague, Jane. She was standing beside me and heard it too."

~

I immediately drove to a colleague's house after school and explained what the assistant principal had revealed. I wanted to call Jane while Deanna was with me so that she could witness the conversation and help me decide how to proceed.

Deanna looked up the number and called Jane.

"Hi Jane, this is Deanna," she said. "I have Gail Lynn here with me. She is quite upset. The assistant principal shared some information with her and we both are finding it hard to believe. Gail Lynn wanted to ask you about it. Actually, the assistant principal told her to ask you. Is it okay if I put you on speakerphone?"

Jane agreed.

"Hi, Jane," I began. For the next ten minutes, we exchanged pleasantries and asked about each other's families. Then I got to the point. "I'm sorry to put you on the spot like this, but, well, the assistant principal shared some things with me in private and told me to confirm them with you if I didn't believe her. I'm having a hard time believing her." Laughing, I continued. "I have a few questions I want to ask you."

"Okay, what are your questions?" Jane replied.

"Well, it sounds really silly and I find it hard to believe, but the assistant principal told me that you were part of a conversation where the principal called me a witch."

Jane laughed. "I wasn't PART of the conversation, but I was standing there when the principal called you a witch. For whatever reason, you really have her scared."

"Can you tell me more about what she said and the conversation? I mean, I don't understand any of it and what brought that up or why she would think such a thing."

"I only caught part of it," said Jane. "She was complaining about her sprained ankle and wearing that boot thing. She looked at me and said she thinks you are a witch and placed a spell on her. She thinks that is why she fell off a ladder over the weekend."

My mouth fell open as I sat there at Deanna's kitchen table. I couldn't believe what I heard. Deanna jumped into the conversation with some questions to try and clarify any miscommunication. Jane continued.

"She said Gail is a witch. I guess because of where you live Gail. She said Lily Dale is full of witches. Funny thing is, she told us that she's been to Lily Dale for readings before, so she must not be that frightened of witches," she chuckled.

I thanked Jane and we said goodbye. Deanna sat and stared at me in disbelief. Neither of us knew what to say next, so we laughed hysterically.

"That woman has a problem," Deanna said.

"I think I have to call the EEOC," I decided.

"I think you should. What do you have to lose?"

"Nothing but more harassment, I guess. I've made it this far, and besides, it's not long before I leave for Hawaii for the summer."

I did as the assistant principal advised and called the EEOC. I explained the situation with my health and fighting

Lyme disease for the past four years. I explained Lily Dale, the spiritual community where I live, and my beliefs about holistic healing, and then I described the various accounts of the principal bullying me. They took down my information and told me to gather documentation and fax it to them.

That night I spent hours writing down notes and adding sticky notes to my medical records to send in. I called my friend Darlene to let her know what I was doing and asked if there was anything else she remembered that I should add.

"I can't believe she called you a witch," Darlene chuckled. "Why does she even go to Lily Dale herself if she really believes you all are witches?"

"She probably goes to Lily Dale because she needs healing, just like so many other people who come there. Sadly, she just doesn't recognize it."

~

That night as I was looking at the staff's End of Year Checklist, I stopped and froze in fear at the sudden realization that I was going to fly out to Hawaii on Thursday, BUT the last day of school had been changed to Friday this year. I became overwhelmed with anxiety. Pacing the floor in my living room, I called Darlene and explained the situation.

"Just use your sick days. Go talk to the superintendent, explain your situation, and you'll be fine. Your health is what matters. Whether you do your things with your oil stuff or see a doctor, it shouldn't matter. It's still your health."

Restless all night, the next day I called the school administration office first thing in the morning and spoke to one of the secretaries. I explained I would be taking the last two days of school off for health reasons and that I was going away for the summer for treatment. She wished me well and suggested that I might want to meet with the interim superintendent so that she knew why I was taking time off.

152

"Our interim superintendent, Ms. Rootabaga, she doesn't know anything about your battle with the Lyme disease. Just explain it to her and if she has any questions, many of us here know you and can explain the circumstances. We want you back healthy!" The secretary made it sound easy, yet my fear was growing.

The following Friday when I signed in at the administration office, I was brought back right away to see Ms. Rootabaga. She greeted me kindly and invited me to sit. I introduced myself, told her a quick history of my position and seventeen years with the school, and then gave her my history of struggles with Lyme disease for the past four years. She was kind, sympathetic, and shared what little she knew of Lyme disease. Then I explained my beliefs about natural healing and that I was going away and was taking off the following Thursday afternoon and Friday to leave for a summer healing journey out of the states. I explained my fear of having to explain to the principal since many of our interactions caused such great stress that I often ended up in the emergency room.

"What do you need from me?" Ms. Rootabaga asked. "I appreciate you coming in to explain your situation, but how can I help you?"

"I'm afraid to tell the principal that I won't be in school for the last two half days. I know I don't have to explain my health to anyone, and that I *can* just put in for a substitute. But I'm not sure how to handle it. If I put in for a substitute, it will cost the district more money. But the aide in my classroom could cover my absence for those few hours and save the district money." I had everything thought out and taken care of so that it wouldn't cause harm to anyone.

"All of my duties are complete as far as preparing the classroom for summer vacation. I even have my report cards done. Thursday morning is only three hours with students, and the aide could read a few books and then take them outside for a field day before dismissal at 11:30 am. Then

Friday, students only come in for an hour for their report cards, and then they are dismissed."

I hesitated to ask. "Can you ask the principal if she wants a substitute or the aid to cover my class? I know it sounds silly, but we butt heads. Ever since her first year when she embarrassed me and brought me to tears in front of my students, we just haven't gotten along. I've asked for a transfer to another school in the district, but so far, it just hasn't worked out because of my illness. I have come so far in getting my health back. I don't want another confrontation with her."

I sat with my head down, knowing how silly it sounded to be afraid to talk to my boss, but I also knew that healing and getting my life back was in sight. I did not want to compromise my progress.

Ms. Rootabaga sat back in her chair and looked at me with a smile. Playing with a pencil, contemplating what to say next, she took a deep breath. "I'll speak to the principal," she agreed. "As for your health, I truly hope you get the help you need. I've heard horrible things about Lyme disease. When you return, I would hope that at some point you and the principal could try to get back on track. She's your boss and you need to be able to communicate with her. You have my blessing. Now go get well, and I'll see you in September."

She stood and reached out her hand to me, and I took it. It felt more like a hug than a handshake. I knew she was empathetic to my years of struggle.

"Thank you," I said. "Really. Thank you for your understanding. Not many people get it." I was choked up by her compassion.

"One more thing," she added as I walked away. "Send me an email about our discussion so that I have it in writing for your file."

"I will," I promised. "This weekend."

Come Sunday, I began the email and briefly outlined our conversation. I was careful not to say too much that was personal and would be in my file for anyone to read. I described my intentions for a summer healing journey and how I was going away for holistic healing to get my health back and my life back. I wrote that I looked forward to teaching in September when I would be healthy again. I thanked her again and sent it off. I was relieved and actually looked forward to my last week of school and to saying goodbye to my students and celebrating with them. We had successfully completed the year.

~

On Monday, I floated through the workday in a kind of ecstasy, singing through the hallways and smiling at everyone I passed. I did get a few sideways glances and frowns, no surprise of course. During lunchtime, I stayed in my classroom to eat and catch up on email, and that's when I found the response from the interim superintendent. I was baffled by her words.

> June 19, 2017
> Gail,
> In order to approve your days, we will need a doctor's note.
> Ms. Rootabaga

Words screamed in my head, *WHAT HAPPENED?*

I told her I didn't see doctors anymore and that I use only holistic healing for treatments.

She gave me her blessing. She wished me well! Why *this sudden change of heart?*

Angry over this new attack on my beliefs, I became enraged at this sudden hostility towards me. I had gone to this interim superintendent out of courtesy, told her everything including that I did not see doctors for treatment since I used alternative healing modalities for my healthcare. She even gave me her blessing.

I called my union rep immediately for advice. I repeated the whole story. The email, the request for a doctor's note, explained that I do not see a doctor, and described my trip for the alternative treatments.

"What am I supposed to do?" I spat out. "Send her a note from the shaman that I'm going to see?" Panic and anxiety arose in me.

"I guess so," the union rep said half-jokingly. Someone from HR told her not to approve the days, so she's asking for a doctor's note. I don't know what to tell you. I guess you have a choice to make. If you leave, you'll have to face the consequences."

"Face what consequences? What do you mean?" I was furious. "They'll *fire* me? Are you saying I have to see a doctor in order to use my sick days? As a spiritualist, my beliefs do not involve traditional Western medicine treatments anymore. I do not use any kind of treatment from doctors or pharmaceuticals. I haven't for over three years now. They can't make me see a doctor, can they? Good grief, this is America, the land of freedom, of choice!"

"Gail, the superintendent is just saying you have to provide a doctor's' note in order for them to approve your leave," he repeated.

"This is ridiculous. We both know the last two half days with students are all games and fun. I have all my duties completed. I'm going away to work on my health. If it were someone else, we both know that this wouldn't be an issue. Another colleague of mine is taking the last day of school off and *he's* not getting this kind of harassment. It's not fair, and you know it!"

"I don't know what to tell you. You have a choice to make."

"I'll send in a health excuse from a shaman when I get there!" I wanted to slam the phone down and let him hear my fury, but with cell phones, there's just a simple "click". My mind screamed of injustices and discrimination. I thought of my son fighting in the military, fighting for American Freedoms.

Where's my freedom? I was becoming angrier by the minute. My mind screamed. *I have the right to my spiritual beliefs and the health practices I choose.*

As the day came closer to when I would be leaving, more emails went back and forth between the superintendent, the union representative, and me. I wasn't about to change my plans. My health was important, and no one was going to stop me. I tried my best to get through the day without any confrontations. I pictured only great health in my mind and even ignored the last email of the day. I left promptly at 3:15 and cheered myself onward. I only had one more day to get through.

~

I woke up Wednesday, my last day before leaving, eager for the day. I put the troubling thoughts out of my mind. I was determined to stay on track, determined to keep my health a priority, determined to make this last day with my students the best day possible.

Although this school year began with me ready to throw in the towel, as my last attempt to make it through, we, my students and I, had finished the year successfully. And as it always was on the last day with students, I was teary-eyed, from the beginning of the day 'til dismissal. I had spent months caring for them and molding their lives. Ten months of not just teaching them academics but teaching them about life and compassion and caring for each other. I had pushed them to do better than they thought possible. I know I made mistakes through the year, yes, I met frustration with anger at times. I may even have been mean and incorrigible at times, but at the heart of my teaching was someone who had been in their shoes many times, feeling lost and unloved myself. I wanted my students to keep pushing through the tough times.

157

I wanted them to give it their all and know that they could BE, DO, and HAVE anything if they were determined.

As students arrived that morning, I told them to gather their latest book that they wrote and bring it to the carpet to share with a friend. I was just about to head to the carpet with my own piece of writing to share with them when the phone rang. It was the school secretary telling me that the principal and the director of elementary education wanted to meet with me at 2:00 pm and that if I wanted a union representative to attend with me, to call for one.

I immediately sent a message to the president of the teacher's union who promptly responded.

My heart began to race at the thought of this meeting. I wondered what they had planned. The secretary couldn't tell me what the meeting was about, so it seemed to be sort of a secret. Standing there at my desk, I was suddenly embraced by one of my students.

"Why do you look like you're going to cry, Ms. Gail?"

I shook my head, laughed, and said I was going to miss them all. I wanted to change the thoughts running through my head. I didn't want to concern myself with some stupid meeting. I didn't want anything to take away from this last day with my students.

"Come on, let's go to the carpet. I want to hear the latest stories everyone wrote." I tried to muster up some excitement.

Sitting with my students, I shared a piece of writing that I wrote the night before. It was a one-page story about overcoming obstacles. It was about being afraid I was going to die from the Lyme disease a few years back and how I never gave up. I wrote about going to Hawaii to get better. Then I told them that it was our last day together and that I was leaving on a plane the next morning to get treatment for my health. I asked them to write me a story that I could read while I was on the plane. Then I asked who wanted to share their latest story.

"Me, me!" they all shouted. It made my heart happy to see them excited about being authors. They too were on the way to becoming writers, to becoming heroes in their own life.

"Ms. Gail, I dedicated my book to you," said one little boy. "Can I read it to you?"

My eyes welled up with tears. I couldn't stop them from spilling over.

Listening to all their thoughts and feelings and life stories that they had written down on paper filled my heart with love and pride for what they had accomplished. It had been quite a year. I wasn't there for them when they started in September, I was wanting to give up. But here I was now, not wanting to leave them. At that moment, they became my pride and joy.

For a while, I was angry with my friend Deanna. She had yelled at me in the hospital and then yelled at me when I wanted to give up and apply for disability. She pushed me to keep going, and perhaps it was that push that gave me the determination that I needed. I guess that was what I tried to do for my students, to push them so that they could see what I had seen, that their strength, their beauty, their ability to do anything was there if they put their mind to it.

Throughout the rest of the day, students randomly came up to hug me. "I'm going to miss you," they said, "you'll get better, Ms. Gail."

Then Jazzy, a sweet little girl with beautiful eyes and curly hair, came up to me. She handed me her story. "Ms. Gail," she whispered. "You're my inspiration. I'm going to miss you. Thank you for teaching us that we can use writing to solve our problems. Thank you for the rocks you gave us. I care about you, Ms. Gail."

The dam burst open and tears flowed down my cheeks. We hugged and then I called for all the students to gather their stories and meet me at the carpet. They saw my tears. "Hey y'all," one student yelled out. "Ms. Gail needs a group hug!"

~

I sat there on a tiny little chair looking at each of their faces, feeling overwhelmed with emotion. "Before I leave," I began, "I want you to know how proud I am of each of you. Sometimes learning can be hard. Sometimes the lessons don't make sense to us. I get it. Even as an adult, life lessons can be hard. We make mistakes. We get things wrong sometimes. But we have to keep going. So, remember, when faced with something that seems difficult, whether it's math or reading or something at home in your family; stay positive. Be the positive side of the battery that gives positive energy to others and before you know it, everything will light up!

"Ask your brain for help. Ask your heart to show you how to solve the problem. When you use your heart and kindness, everything will work out."

I called each student up for a hug then asked for their stories. I explained to them that I would read them while sitting on the airplane flying tomorrow morning. I said my goodbyes then turned to the aide to give her directions for the remaining time with students. Then I left for the meeting.

Deep breaths calmed me down on the walk to the conference room. The union president was already talking with the principal and the director of elementary education when I walked in.

As soon as I sat down, the principal began.

"The superintendent denied the days off, Gail, and I'm expecting you to be here these last two days of school. As you know, you are being transferred to teach pre-kindergarten next year so I am expecting you to attend some professional development classes over the summer to help prepare you to teach our pre-kindergarten students in the fall."

I looked at her and then at the union president. I expected him to step in and say something about her

160

comment and having to take summer classes, but he just kept writing in his notebook, trying to look busy.

I took another deep breath and tried to keep my cool. I wasn't about to let her push my buttons as she had so often in the past. I kept picturing Hawaii in my thoughts.

"Excuse me," I said quietly. "Summer vacation is just that, a vacation. Teachers are not expected, nor required to take classes over the summer. It is an option if we would like to. I am going away for the summer to work on my health. I have lost a lot of work over the past four years due to my health and I am going to do something to rid the illness once and for all. I will not be in the states over the summer."

I could see the anger rising in her face as she looked back and forth between the Director of Education and me. She leaned in close to me, raised her hand, and pointed a finger at me. "You were denied those days off," she hissed. "You are expected to be in your classroom tomorrow and I am *directing* you to attend a summer workshop–"

The director of education cut her off mid-sentence. "Gail, of course, you don't *have* to attend any summer workshops, but we would like you to. You have taught many different grade levels, and this will be new for you, so it would be good to get some background on our PreK program for students," she stated calmly.

"As director of elementary education," I replied, "you know my teaching capabilities. Especially since you requested me as your own son's teacher just a few years ago, before I was struck with this awful illness. You of all people know my teaching strengths. I ran my own daycare before I started teaching. I have taught kindergarten, first grade, third grade, and fourth grade. I've raised three children. I am quite capable of successfully teaching four-year-old students in our PreK program come fall."

I turned to the principal and continued. "Furthermore, you cannot give me a *directive* to attend anything over the summer per our teacher's contract. So, I'm not sure why we are having this meeting."

"Gail," the director jumped in. "We are letting you know of the change in your placement, that's all."

"I've already been informed that I was being moved. But that is usually done in a letter anyway. Have you called in other teachers to tell them of their change in placement also, or just me? Because I can document this as continued harassment."

"Well, we also want to know if you plan on coming into school tomorrow," asked the director. "We need to know for the sake of a substitute."

"I met with the superintendent. She approved of me going away AND wished me well, actually. Quite kind of her. She explained to me that she would handle the rest with the principal. I won't be in tomorrow, as I told the superintendent. I'm going away to work on my health. I am protected by HIPPA laws and I do not need to provide you the details of my health situation. My classroom duties are complete and here is my checklist of duties marked off." I slid the paper across the table to the director.

The principal was unable to control herself any longer. She stood in a fury as the chair screeched back away from the table. She pointed her finger at me and raised her voice. "I'm so disappointed in you, Gail. You should be here to attend summer workshops for your new grade level. You were told by the HR department that you don't have permission for your sick days, so I'm expecting you to be in your classroom the last two days of school."

I leaned forward and tried not to lose control. "You're disappointed in *me*?" I hissed. "Excuse me, but the acting superintendent *did* give me permission. And from my understanding, she was told by others in the admin office afterward *not* to give me permission. You can't stop me from taking care of my health. That's discrimination."

I looked over at the union representative for support, but he did not stir. Instead, he continued to sit with his eyes focused down at his notebook, so I continued. "Ms. Rootabaga gave me approval and asked me to put it in writing for her. I have a flight. I do not need to explain my health issues to you. It is not your business how I treat my health conditions. I have rights! I shouldn't have to choose between my health and my job! Lastly, my year-end classroom duties are complete. I secured a substitute just in case you wanted one. Everything is done. Here's the key to my classroom. I'll be back in August healthy and ready to begin. I'll be successful in the new grade level like I've been every year I am moved!"

I left my key on the table and walked out of the conference room. It was 3:15 pm and the school day was over. I headed to my classroom, arranged the desktop for the sub to find everything easily, then wrote a short note on the whiteboard for my students to read in the morning:

June 22, 2017
Dear Students,
You are amazing authors! Keep writing great stories!
I am on my way to get healthy again. Have a great summer!
Come see me in September!
Love,
Ms. Gail

I shut the lights off and walked out to my car where I sat sad and angry while I gathered my thoughts. It didn't make much difference if they fired me if staying meant I would wind up back in the hospital every three months. I had to ask myself what was more important, my job or my health.

Angry thoughts flashed through my mind. "Don't I matter?" I screamed out as I drove home. No one responded.

I parked in front of my house and ran in long enough to grab my suitcases and flight itinerary and get back into my car. I had an early flight in the morning and since my friend Denise made a last-minute decision to attend the conference and visit her sisters on the Big Island as well, she invited me to sleep at her house. She couldn't get on my flight as it was already full, so she had to get up earlier and drive to Toronto. Her fiancé was going to drop me off at the Buffalo airport at 5:00 am.

I was all distraught when I arrived at her house. Between the time I left school and Denise's house, the school administration office had called twice. Afraid they were going to try to stop me, I didn't answer. I was even more afraid of ending up back in the hospital. That was the pattern after a heated debate with the school administrator. I explained everything to Denise and her fiancé.

"Make an appointment to see a doctor when you get to Maui," Denise said. She was always so matter-of-fact and had an answer for even the most difficult problems. "I'll go with you!" she exclaimed.

Even though she didn't understand my fear of doctors and Western medicine, I was grateful she had decided to join me for the ten days on Maui. I was privately praying for her company. I wanted her to escort me to Hawaii because secretly, I was scared of going alone. I had never traveled by myself and The Fear Miser was threatening to hurt me.

I spent a restless night at her house worrying about my job. I could not afford to be fired, but I couldn't keep going the way I was, either. The words of Doc Munshi resonated in my head. "Once you have Lyme disease, you will always have it," he had told me. "Stress kills people." But I was about to prove him wrong. I was going to prove everyone wrong in the Lyme community and Hawaii was going to help me. I just didn't know how.

~

On the morning of June 22, 2017, I boarded a plane at 5:35 am. Although I had little sleep from worrying all night, I felt wide-awake. Alive. My heart was pounding as thoughts began to race through my mind, questioning myself as to whether this healing journey was indeed the right choice. But there was also another voice in me somewhere that urged me to keep going and never turn back.

Follow your heart, I heard.

Taking my seat on the plane, I turned on my iPod and began listening to Wayne Dyer. His soothing voice settled me.

Wayne, I prayed, *I am so afraid. Am I doing the right thing? You were sick, yet you healed the Leukemia in your body. You have helped millions of people heal. Please help me. God, am I doing the right thing? Please help me.*

My throat tightened as I held back the tears. The plane gave a sudden jerk as it began moving away from the gate. Fighting the fear that was trying to take over, I texted my friend, Mary.

I'm scared, say a little prayer for me.

Feeling anxious, I turned and looked at the empty seat next to me and then the stranger with his head leaning against the window. I envied his peace. I shut my eyes again and spoke to God. *Why didn't Denise get on the same plane as me?* I took a deep breath and tried focusing on the sound of Wayne Dyer's voice coming through my headphones.

Feeling the bumps as we taxied to the runway, I took a deep breath and reassured myself that it would all be okay. The engines engaged and roared as we prepared for takeoff. I clutched the armrests, bracing for the speed that was coming. The cabin vibrated with the effort of the engines and then…everything stopped! An eerie feeling came over me. The engines were hushed, and all forward movement ceased.

Panic came over me. I removed the earplugs to hear the husky voice coming over the loudspeakers.

"Ladies and gentlemen, this is your pilot speaking. We seem to be having some technical difficulty with our control panel. We are getting in touch with maintenance and will keep you informed. The voice boomed confidence, yet every part of my being was afraid.

Fear. Worry. Panic. It all washed over me.

I texted Mary again.

    I'M SCARED. PROBLEMS WITH PLANE.

She responded.

    Gail, stay in the vortex.

I was angry at her lack of concern. I texted her again.

    REALLY MARY? THERE'S PROBLEMS
    WITH CONTROL PANEL.

She texted back.

    Something good is going to come of this.

    Keep me posted.

The pilot's voice boomed over the PA system again. "Ladies and gentlemen, we are going to have to head back to the gate for maintenance to come on board. There's going to be about an hour time delay, and we will be making some changes so that everyone can make their flight connections. We will keep you posted."

I texted Mary again.

    HOUR DELAY! PLANE PROBLEMS! OMG
    MARY! WHAT THE HELL DO YOU THINK
    IS GOING ON?

Fear coursed through my body.

As we pulled up to the gate, the pilot spoke to us once again. "Ladies and gentlemen, we apologize for any inconvenience, but we are going to need to reroute a few passengers in order to make flight connections. We need the following passengers to grab their luggage and come to the front of the plane: Gail Lynn–" I didn't wait to hear the rest of the names, I just got up and off the plane in anxious confusion. The passenger from the seat beside me was right behind me on our way off the plane.

"If you two will follow me back inside, we will get you taken care of. It looks like you both are going to Maui, and we need to reroute you in order for you to make all your flight connections," explained the agent.

I turned and looked at the stranger next to me. He was tall and thin, with day-old facial hair and an unimpressed look on his face. His skin was dark from time spent in the sun. He had beautiful green eyes that looked down at me in a peaceful manner. Something shifted at that moment, and suddenly I was excited again about my trip to Maui.

I struck up a conversation with him while the agent got our itineraries together.

"You're going to Maui, too?" I asked. "Have you ever been there before?"

The stranger turned and looked at me with tender eyes and nodded.

The agent handed us our itineraries and said we had plenty of time before we needed to board if we wanted to get breakfast. A million thoughts sped through my mind.

"You have? You've been to Maui before?" I asked eagerly. "This is my first time. I'm going to find new healing techniques. I have Lyme disease and I'm going to the Hay House Writer's Workshop to learn about writing and healing. Have you heard of it before? Have you ever heard of Hay House?"

Again, he looked at me with a sideways glance and nodded. "Yes," he spoke. "I live down the road from there."

"Shut up, really?" I laughed. "You live on Maui? That's great! Wayne Dyer is a writer who used to present at these conferences, but he died. Have you ever heard of Wayne Dyer? He was a great man and a great writer. His work changed my life."

The stranger put his hand to his chin contemplatively. "Yes," he said. "I knew him. He was a patient of mine."

"Seriously?" I exclaimed. "You met Wayne Dyer? You were a doctor of his? I was just on the plane listening to his podcast, and you, his doctor, were sitting next to me! That's crazy!"

Beyond ecstatic now, I continued babbling while he stood politely listening.

"Wayne understood this," I said. "I've been sick for over four years and I'm just beginning to learn how disease enters the body and how we can heal naturally with alternative health modalities. How did he die? He of all people knew HOW TO HEAL. I'm writing a book about healing. I've had Lyme disease for over four years now, and it's been so bad at times that I literally wanted to die and tried to find ways to end my life. But I'm getting better. I think I get it now. I think I finally know how to heal this once and for all. The funny thing is, I may lose my job at the expense of taking this journey to get my health back."

I was over-the-top excited to be standing there speaking with a doctor who once treated Wayne Dyer, my spiritual mentor, my hero. I realized I was rambling and stopped to look over at this stranger who was put into my life. Then Spirit gave me an insight. I was shown an image of Wayne Dyer, sad with a broken heart.

"Never mind," I said. "I know how he died. He had a broken heart."

I didn't tell the stranger why I thought this. I didn't want to tell him that I spoke to Wayne often in my head or sometimes even out loud. My heart felt Wayne's heart right then, like one who knew, like one who walked that same mile.

I looked down at the stranger's long feet in his flip-flops. Suddenly another image flashed through my mind. The scene was from another era. The feet were similar, although the road upon which he was standing was dry and dusty. I shook my head to clear my thoughts then looked back up into the man's eyes.

He looked at me strangely. Feeling uncomfortable with his stare, I continued talking. "I do not believe in traditional Western medicine anymore. One doctor told me I was sick because of the flip-flops I was wearing and that a woman my age should be wearing supportive shoes."

My eyes were still drawn to his feet. He was a doctor, a few years older than I was, and there he was in flip-flops. I laughed and kept rambling until he interrupted.

"Shall we head to our gate?" he asked.

Nodding, I began to walk alongside him, continuing my ramble. "I turned to alternative healing modalities a few years ago. Nobody believes we can heal using other means, I guess. I don't know why. But the school where I work is asking for a doctor's note even though I told them I don't see doctors anymore. I don't have a doctor's note. My union rep told me the school is going to try to fire me."

Tears began welling up as I explained my dilemma. I'm not sure why I was telling this man my life story. Perhaps it was his compassionate eyes or his lips that smiled ever so slightly.

I looked up to see that we were at our gate and found a spot to sit. I lowered my voice even more, trying to suffocate the feelings that had been building in my chest. "The school is making me choose between my job and my health," I went on. The tightness in my chest rose to my throat as I held back tears. I reprimanded myself for getting caught up in emotions with a total stranger. *Don't cry, Gail. Keep it in. Don't let it out.*

"Do you mean to tell me that your employer is going to fire you because you don't have a doctor's note?" he asked.

"Yes," I said. "I stopped seeing my doctor over a year ago. I was only going for consultations and tests. I use alternative healing modalities like essential oils for antibiotics and inflammation and Reiki and EFT. I'm sorry. I've just had too many doctors throw pills at me and not help get to the root of what was causing the illness. Can you believe a doctor told me I was sick because of the flip-flops I was wearing? That's neither a good doctor nor a good healthcare system. I've been so sick for so long, so I turned to alternative healing. And that's why I'm here and writing and looking for a shaman."

I remembered the union president's comment that someone in the administration told her not to approve my leave. "The school superintendent lied," I told him everything. "She gave me permission to come, but then the HR office said she didn't. And because I couldn't give them a doctor's note, they are going to try to fire me. Because of my beliefs that we can heal naturally, because of the spiritual community where I live, I am being harassed."

Not wanting this stranger to see the tears starting to form, I looked away. I loved teaching. I was proud of being a good teacher. Over the years, I had many administrators and colleagues who had requested me to be their child's teacher. I knew I was good, but they wanted me to think otherwise. I hated feeling weak. I hated crying. I hated that my employer could reduce me to tears. I hated that they wanted to control me, my health, and my life.

"I'm a doctor," the stranger said. "Let's talk. That took a lot of courage for you to leave. We can have a consultation in my office when we get to Maui, and I can write you a doctor's note. Tell me about the Lyme disease."

He opened his wallet and handed me his business card. I looked at him then at the card. I was finally speechless. My mouth was open, and my mind was boggled as I searched for the right words. I didn't know whether to laugh or cry.

The name on the business card was foreign. "Thank you Dr. Hosh...mond Paj...bak...koli," I stammered. "You probably just saved me my job. Sorry, I know I just botched your name. How do you say it correctly?"

"It's okay," he said. "Just call me Dr. P."

"Okay, Dr. P. Thank you for listening to me. I like your name though. Where is it from? Where's your family from? My father's side of the family is from Sicily, so I understand people botching up pronunciation. My maiden name is Mongitore. People have messed it up so badly before and called me Ms. Mongaloid." I laughed.

"It doesn't matter where I am from," Dr. P said with a wave of his hand and a discouraged look on his face.

"I don't really care where you're from," I continued. "I believe that I am One with everyone. I believe we all are from the same Source which makes us all in the same family."

He turned to face me again and spoke with a most gentle voice. "My name is Persian. I am from Iran." He paused as if anticipating some kind of reaction.

I shrugged. For a split second, I thought about how the news portrayed Iran, but this man in front of me was nothing like that. He felt familiar to me.

He stood and zipped open his duffle bag, pulling out a pack of cigarettes. "I need to have a smoke before boarding. I'm going to leave my little carry-on right here. Will you be here? We can talk more about the Lyme disease after my cigarette."

"Yes, I'm not going anywhere," I said. As he walked away, the dam that had been holding back the flood finally released, and down my cheeks the rivers flowed unchecked once again. I placed my hand on his little black duffle bag, and something stirred in my heart. I looked at the people seated across from me. I could see their thoughts as if they were floating above their heads in bubbles. The strangest feeling came over me.

"What's happening?" I whispered to Wayne again. I felt the response come with a shiver up my spine.

You can see clearly now.

"Yes," I whispered. "I can. I can see clearly now." And then the people seated across from me who were looking at me with sympathetic eyes had thought bubbles over their heads. I could see their thoughts as if a cartoonist had drawn their words in a cloud over their heads.

"Poor girl, must be she had a death in the family."

"Maybe she's getting divorced."

"Aw, poor thing, she's crying, I hope she's okay."

I could feel the emotions of the family seated across from me as they stared at me. I wanted to look at them, but I couldn't. I wanted them to see *me*, not my sorrow or shame, but the hope that this doctor had just given me; hope that there *IS* good in the world. There IS compassion in our world. We *DO* live in a kind world.

I pulled out my journal to document this moment. As I thumbed through the pages to find my place, I saw the last entry that I had begun just hours earlier while I waited to board the plane.

> *Thursday, June 22, 2017*
> *Divine Love*
> *I am the light*
> *Dear Wayne,*
> *Thank you for being in my life. Thank you for being a light to all humanity! You have made a difference in my life! May I carry the torch, the light, and continue your legacy of helping serve the World of humanity bringing divine love, helping souls to experience divine love, BE divine love, express divine love.*
> *Thank you, thank you, thank you, Wayne.*

I turned the page and continued to write.

> *June 22 ...*
> *Sickness/illnesses are a result of fears, thoughts, and emotions that are merely expressing themselves in our cells. Fear and worry attack our cells. As Wayne says, "Change your thoughts, change your life." Change your beliefs into what you want to manifest. I used to think I would never amount to anything, but today, with your light and the light of any spiritual teachers around me, I now understand I AM worthy, I AM loved. I AM all that I am, that I choose to be. I am so grateful for you, Wayne Dyer. I am changing the way, no, I HAVE changed the way I look at things and I will continue to manifest, I allow all good things and blessing to now come into my life! I AM entitled. I DESERVE great happiness and great health, great wealth, great friendships, and a great journey for the next 50 years! Light converts darkness into light —*

that's alchemy! We all are light! Thank you, Wayne!
THIS is why I had to come to Hawaii for healing:
writing, yes, compassion, yes, empathy, yes.

~

I spent eighteen hours traveling to Maui with Dr. P and discussing Lyme disease – the symptoms, causes, treatments, and beliefs. I gleaned more knowledge and information in our talks than I had over the past four years with various doctors, hospitals, and specialists in western New York. When we finally arrived in Maui, we got our luggage and walked outside.

"Do you need a ride somewhere?" he asked.

I looked up at him in wonder. "Thank you, but you have done so much already. I am meeting my friend, Denise here at the airport. She arrived here before me and should be getting our rental car right now."

I dropped my things and went up to Dr. P and hugged him tightly. I held on for what seemed like quite a long time. I didn't want to let go. This stranger I just met was going out of his way to help me. My old pattern and lack of self-worth still caused many questions to formulate in my mind. When I finally let go and stepped back, I looked up into his beautiful green eyes and wondered if my embrace had made him uneasy. Again, he simply gave me a warm smile and thanked me in return. My heart felt full, and a warm, fuzzy feeling came over me.

"Thank you for being my Earth angel, Dr. P. I don't know how this all happened, how the Universe put you in my life when I needed a doctor's note, but I am so incredibly grateful." My eyes welled up with tears as we said goodbye.

"I'll be in touch in the morning," Dr. P smiled, turned, and walked away.

Behind me, I heard Denise ask, "Who was that?"

"A doctor!" I said. "You're never going to believe this! We were pulled off the plane together in Buffalo and rerouted to be traveling companions the whole way to Maui! Can you believe it? We had a consultation, and I'm going to meet him again tomorrow and he's going to write an excuse for me and send it to the school! I feel like I'm in the twilight zone, Denise! There really are angels looking out for me!" Half laughing, half crying, I rambled on in seemingly nonsensical sentences.

"WHAT? Seriously? See! God always has our back."

I kept repeating the story as we walked toward the rental cars. A doctor. The plane. Wayne's doctor. The Lyme disease. A doctor's note for the school. The beautiful stranger who may have saved my job. It was too perfect to believe.

We got our rental car and made our way to the condo we had rented in Ka'anapali, and I explained the whole story to her yet again.

"Wow, Gail," she said. "We kept saying you needed to see a doctor when you got to Maui and look what happened. You manifested a doctor."

"That's all that was on my mind last night as I fell asleep was getting a doctor's note. You kept drilling that into my head about finding a doctor, and BAM! The Universe provides! You know that the Bible says, 'Ask and you shall receive.' Maybe there really is a God listening to me after all."

The next morning, Dr. P faxed a note to the school to excuse me for my absences, which freed me to focus on the healing journey I had begun. No more stressing about losing my job. I had stood up to the school and stood up against the system that was not supporting me. I had finally stood up for myself. "No more fear now Gail," I told myself. "Get the answers you came here for."

In my greatest time of need, I had spoken out fervently, asking to be led to a doctor to get a note for my employer. The Universe, my angels, and God had supplied me with a doctor who wrote an excuse so that I wouldn't lose my job. I needed help. I asked for help. By following my heart, I received a great gift and could now continue with my healing.

> *"Ask and it will be given to you; seek and you will find; knock and the door will be opened to you."*

~Matthew 7:7 (NIV)

~10~

The Gift of Love

That morning, while sitting at the Hay House Writer's Workshop, I was hanging on every word of CEO Reid Tracy as he welcomed us all to the annual conference. It startled me when my phone went off with an email notification. I had forgotten to put it on silent. I quieted my phone and looked at the email: Office of Dr. Paj'Bakoli. I quickly opened it and saw a few statements followed by an attachment.

"Denise!" I turned my phone for her to see. "Dr. P sent me the doctor's note! LOOK!"

She leaned in to see. "No more worries now, Gail Lynn," she whispered. "You're safe."

~

I had a hard time focusing for the next several minutes. My mind traveled from Wayne Dyer to the school district that threatened to fire me to the realization that the stranger next to me on the plane was put into my life to assist me.

"Am I dreaming?" I whispered aloud. Often talking to myself, I sometimes wondered if the words came out for all to hear or if they were spoken in my head only. Again,

Denise leaned over to me. "Everything always works out," she reassured me.

I chuckled as I remember the last two years attending the Ester Hicks conferences. Denise and I were sending each other videos daily to inspire one another, often mimicking the words of Abraham Hicks, "Everything is always working out for me."

The rest of the day my mind was in and out of a dreaming state. On one hand, I began to see the power of creating our life by our thoughts and words and reveled in the tropical paradise Maui was offering me. On the other hand, I kept fearing something was looming, something bad was going to happen. My thoughts were like a pendulum that kept swinging back and forth between something really good that just happened and the fear that something really bad was going to happen. Then, I contemplated Dr. P and the magic of him appearing in my life.

Later that evening, Dr. P called. "Did you get the email? My secretary sent you the letter she faxed to your school."

"YES! I did!" I said. "Oh, Dr. P, I am so, so grateful for you. I cannot tell you much I appreciate you. How was your day back to work after all your traveling?"

"Oh good, good."

"Will I get to see you again?" Crossing my fingers, I closed my eyes and imagined having dinner with Dr. P and offering my appreciation to him. "Are you free for dinner some night? My treat!" I exclaimed.

"I need to catch up on sleep. My days and nights are confused."

"HUH?" I laughed.

"Never mind. I'll be in touch."

We hung up and I immediately went to tell Denise about our conversation. "I don't know what it is Denise, but I just have this feeling about Dr. P, like...I don't know. It's like he's an old friend or something, someone important that I haven't seen in a long, long time."

We went outside to stroll the beautiful gardens along the pathways that led to the beach. It wasn't long before I was sleepy. "The clock says 8:00 pm," I said, "but my body says, 'You should be sleeping.'"

The following morning, once again I woke up early at 3:00 am, 9:00 am New York time, unable to adjust to the time difference. I used the time to speak to Wayne and write. Daily, my laptop sat with me like a best friend waiting for my thoughts to be recorded. When The Fear Miser started lingering, I began repeating affirmations to hold it at bay.

Over coffee that morning, I confided to Denise. "I felt like I was being followed yesterday. I don't know why, I just have this feeling. Do you think the school sent someone to follow me?"

"You know you are a creator," she reminded me. "Create a different thought. Everything will work out."

That day I continued to meet people from all parts of the world who came to learn about writing, about healing, about incorporating the two into their lives. As I met these new friends, I began to see something in them, a connection of some sort. It was an odd feeling I kept having; I was seeing strangers as either a friend or foe.

I had read so many books about the power of our thoughts and intentions, but trying to implement what I had learned and change old patterns that had accumulated over the past fifty years was difficult. Nonetheless, I forged ahead and wrote affirmations on post-it notes and placed them on my computer, in the bathroom, in the car, and in my journal. I wrote affirmations of love, gratitude, and feeling safe. The feeling of being followed, though, stuck with me.

The following day, more of the same occurred. I woke at 3:00 am, talked with Wayne, and wrote in my manuscript of the Healing Journey to Hawaii and becoming the heroine of my own life. Throughout the day, I concentrated on the daily teachings of the various presenters during the writer's workshop. I ate lunch with authors, energy healers, and practitioners in the healing field. I met others who had battled Lyme disease and other illnesses, and I forged connections that supported my healing process.

Having conversations with others who had faced "mysterious" illnesses and used alternative healing was a tremendous perk of the conference. I was making even greater connections between illnesses and emotions, and not just my own. More and more, I was gathering little puzzle pieces and putting them together to form chunks of a larger picture that gave me much to think about creating our own symptoms, illnesses, and lives in general.

Digging deeper into conversations over lunch, I began to see a pattern of sadness, sorrow, and negative emotions that led up to each person's illness. I documented it all as a theory: resentment, shame, anger, fear, depression, and guilt were the starting point of many illnesses.

Later that evening, Dr. P called again to inquire about my day and how I was feeling. "I had no time to even think about my symptoms, exhaustion, or pain," I told him. "I sat in the warm sand after our classes and floated in the ocean. I think the pain has dissipated."

We made a plan to have dinner the following night. Denise and I would meet him at a little oceanfront restaurant. After hanging up, feeling sleepy, I retired early to my bed to write. I took out my journal and computer and sat them both on the bed. The journal called to me first, so I picked it up and ran my finger over the cover title as I read it.

2017 Allow the Enfolding.

There was a picture of a butterfly on the front cover which fit the theme of my life, transformation. Its beauty settled into my mind's eye, and an image of Wayne Dyer popped into my head. In one of his books, he talked about a monarch butterfly that landed on his finger while the Maui trade winds tried relentlessly to blow it off, but the monarch held fast. The story Wayne tells is of a close friend who passed into the spirit world and was speaking to him through the butterfly that had landed on him. This stuck with me.

I often feel the same way when I see a butterfly or a Cardinal or hear a specific song on the radio. That was how Spirit often brought messages to me from the other side. Like the time when Stevie Nicks came on the radio while I was driving home from work one day. I started singing, "No one knows, how I feel..." Then my friend, Jimmy, who at that moment was in the hospital undergoing surgery, popped into my awareness as if he was present. He was floating, staring at me through the windshield. Then he began to float up through the clouds while waving to me and saying goodbye. I had to pull over.

"What, Jimmy?" I asked, confused.

"Goodbye, Gail," he said. "I'm going. Be there for my sister and my parents. I'm free now."

"NO! Please don't go, Jimmy!" I cried so hard and begged him to stay. I yelled at God, "I don't want this gift!"

At 8:00 am the next morning, his sister called to let me know he was in a coma and asked if I would come put frankincense oil on his head to help heal him. I knew he was already gone, but I went. I stood at the foot of his bed where he was no longer in his body and went through the motions of praying for him to stay along with the rest of his family.

Being clairvoyant wasn't always easy.

~

The image that I saw of the butterfly sparked an inner conversation with Wayne. I closed my eyes and asked him if he had orchestrated everything that happened for me to meet Dr. P. I sent him my most heartfelt gratitude and gushed with love for his part in my summer healing journey to Hawaii.

I sat quietly for a few minutes to contemplate the past few days. I felt fortunate to have crossed paths with Dr. P but still questioned how it all happened. It was a gift from the Universe. Being in Hawaii, meeting Dr. P, all of it was a gift.

Feeling nostalgic, I opened my journal and began reading from the beginning, January 2017, when the enfoldment began. Skimming on to February, I began to read a little slower, taking my time to process what was before me. The words on the pages were about wanting a better life, a healthier life, and the desire to *manifest* things. One entry, in particular, stopped me in my tracks:

February 22, 2017
Reid Tracey, CEO of Hay House, one day we will meet.

"Oh, my God!" I whispered. Then I spoke louder. "THIS… JUST… HAPPENED! JUNE 22!"

Contemplating the events before me, I screamed for Denise to come and see. She came into the bedroom and I held up my journal for her to see.

"Look at the date!" I squealed. "On February 22, I wrote that one day I would meet Reid Tracey, and here, in Maui, June 22, I MET HIM!"

I was beside myself, exuberant with joy. "Is that crazy? How do you explain what's happening to me? Am I going crazy?"

"Gee, Gail Lynn!" she smiled. "You are quite the little manifesting queen!" I jumped on the bed like a child, giggling, as Denise joined in with me. "I told you that you were a little creator. I wonder what's next!"

I flopped down on the bed and stared at Denise. "Doesn't this seem a bit strange?" I asked. "I mean first meeting Dr. P and now seeing how I wrote in my journal months ago about wanting to meet Reid Tracy, and here I am in Maui having just met Reid Tracy!" I waited for an explanation.

Denise just smiled and shrugged and grabbed my hand, pulling me off the bed. "Let's see what we can manifest to eat! I'm starving. The heck with sleep, we can do that next week when we go see Wendy on the Big Island."

Denise was smiling at me mischievously as she searched for something on her phone. As we got into the car, I heard the voice of Ester Hicks speaking, "Everything always works out for me, everything *always* works out for me..." Denise and I joined in, giggling, repeating everything Ester way saying.

Denise drove to the local ABC store. Perusing the aisles, we decided on a few snacks to take back to the condo. It was getting late and our bodies still weren't adjusted to the time change.

~

The next day at the writer's workshop, Reid Tracy introduced another award-winning author. The author shared her story about her two-year-old son who woke up one day and began talking about his life as a famous baseball player. Listening carefully, I waited for a punch line as if it was a joke. Realizing she was telling a true story, I slid to the edge of my seat and poked Denise.

"Can you believe this?" I whispered.

"I know," she said. "Like what we talked about in your kitchen last year."

The memory came to mind instantly. Denise and her fiancé, Brian, were at my house for dinner. After meditation, we sat and talked about visions we had of other lifetimes. The thought had crossed my mind many times before. I used to kid Bryce about a past life we shared. Everyone laughed when I brought it up, so I stopped talking about it. That is until that night meditating with Denise and Brian. Now I wondered aloud as I sat there in Maui. "Denise, maybe Dr. P was in one of my past lives. Maybe that's why he feels so familiar. And if Dr. P was, perhaps Wayne was, too!"

~

Later that evening, the magic of Maui continued as Dr. P, Denise, and I sat watching the sunset from our oceanside table. Something was happening to my heart. I gazed out at the ocean, then at Dr. P, then Denise. Back and forth I watched and listened. As if under the spell of Maui and this man, I sat like a watchful observer of their conversation, wondering if the whole thing was a movie playing on stage somewhere. We were enjoying a magnificent Maui sunset over dinner as if it were a normal daily occurrence. The sky was a painter's palette and became more exquisite as the minutes passed.

Just as the sun kissed the horizon and began to sink into the Pacific, I set my eyes on the stranger beside me who had entered my life. In my mind, I spoke to him.

Who are you? Where did you come from? How did you end up in my life? Was it you that I was supposed to find on this quest and not a shaman? Are you real? Is this real?

Dr. P was not just a thoughtful and compassionate human, he was also strikingly handsome. His high cheekbones and deep-set eyes alluded to some kind of mystery. I sensed that his smile, which appeared every so often, hid secrets of both pleasure and pain. Stealing a glance, I allowed my eyes to soften, then shifting my eyes to his heart, I began to sense his energy field. It felt familiar. My heart secretly whispered to my mind, *I know him.*

Lost in thought, I began to think about a recording I heard of Wayne Dyer. He spoke about a past life regression that he had with a woman, Mira Kelley. He spoke about traveling to the Polynesian islands once before. A spark of light occurred in my mind and shone out as if from a lighthouse. Then, a beam of light went from my heart to Dr. P's heart, and I suddenly became aware of a feeling that was rising in me. Not just gratitude and appreciation for this man, but love, a deep love that felt familiar, comfortable. There were visions of people in my mind, people walking through a dusty village, wearing sheaths of cloth. They were tan, simple, and wore cords around their waists. I heard my name

184

and came back to the present moment, shaking the vision out of my mind.

"That must've been a good little dream you just had there," Denise snickered.

"I'm in a dream right now," I giggled. "Pinch me."
Both Dr. P and Denise chuckled.

After dinner, we strolled along the oceanfront. It still felt oddly familiar walking Ka'anapali Beach where Wayne once lived, where he took his daily swim in the ocean. I was enamored of it all. Darkness fell upon us and the evening sky of glittering diamonds settled in. Torches lit the path. Men who twirled fire batons came onto the beach to entertain tourists.

The beauty of Maui, the chance meeting with Dr. P, and all of the knowledge that I was gaining from the conference workshops were too much. My heart was expanding with each experience and I was so grateful, yet poking at me ever so slightly was fear and the lingering lack of worthiness.

The voice in my head was all too familiar. The Fear Miser was returning. *Who do you think you are,* it echoed. *You don't deserve this. You are nobody. Don't get used to it. You got lucky. It won't last.*

Fear spoke in my mind whenever anything good happened to me. It convinced me I wasn't good enough or worthy. I pushed it right away.

The three of us walked the beach in silence until Denise broke the spell and said we should head home and do our homework for tomorrow's class.

"Ah yes, your class," Dr. P said. "I should let you ladies get home. Well, if you enjoyed this sunset, tomorrow you should come to my house and watch it from there. I live up higher on the mountain and the view is even more breathtaking." He looked at me and then Denise.

"Sure!" I shouted enthusiastically, not waiting for Denise to respond. Chuckling, I turned to her to see if she wanted to see an even more spectacular sunset tomorrow. Of course, she did.

"Really, Dr. P," I said trying to be serious. "Thank you so much for everything. You've been so kind and giving. How do I thank you?"

"No need," he said. "Just come tomorrow. Be my guests. I'll call you after work and give you directions." His quiet disposition was unchanging. He smiled simply as we said goodbye and went our separate ways.

Driving back to the condo, Denise reminded me that we were still without a place to stay the last two nights on Maui. "Remember your bright idea of not booking a room for our last two nights?" she asked. "Have you thought about what part of the island you'd like to explore?"

"Well, Denise," I said. "I have some ideas, but let's see what happens tomorrow."

~

The next day was another full day of learning at the writer's workshop. I took notes and wrote out ideas when one of the authors said that she began picturing in her mind what her final book would look like and then created a book cover that she looked at every day.

I began experimenting with this idea for my own book project. Contemplating images of the island, using the pictures I had taken thus far on Maui, I knew then that I was creating a vision of what my book would be like. I began to wonder if you could visualize a book right into existence if that is what this author did. Then it struck me, might I also be able to visualize a healthy body right into existence as well? Ideas flowed and I began scribbling in my journal. Drawing pictures of stick figures and Maui beaches, I was reminded of the vision boards that I use to create with my friends. *Maybe there is something more to this*, I thought.

After the day of classes, we drove back to the condo and freshened up. Dr. P called and gave us directions to his house. We arrived with a bottle of wine to gift Dr. P for hosting the sunset viewing. As we drove up the driveway, Denise and I were entranced by the magnificence of his property. A large stone Buddha statue greeted us as we passed through the gate. The driveway was lined with palm trees and tropical flowers on both sides.

It looked like heaven. The lawn and gardens were immaculate. The view was indeed breathtaking. Dr. P met us warmly at the entrance to his home.

"Come," he said. "Follow me."

He walked the cobblestone path that led to the covered lanai where even more grandeur awaited us. An infinity pool and hot tub added to the magical setting with the Pacific Ocean and island of Lāna'i in the background. The beauty of the stage set for our evening showcase was like nothing I had ever seen in my life.

I handed Dr. P the bottle of wine, and his face lit up. "Thank you," he said. "You didn't need to bring anything. Choose your seat. The show is about to start. I'll grab some glasses."

I sat there in awe, taking it all in. "Your home is absolutely gorgeous! I've never seen such a beautiful place, Dr. P. Thank you for inviting us here to join you." I looked over at Denise who also sat wide-eyed and happy.

"Yes, thank you Dr. P for sharing your home with us," she said.

"You're welcome," he replied. "It's a shame that more people don't get to see this," he said. "But I don't like large crowds of people, and I don't care to entertain. This, though, is nice."

How does one choose the words to describe the miracle of creation, of the sun and moon and the stars and all that is? A captivating display, a grand, exquisite evening unfolded and truly nothing spoken could have fit the magic felt throughout the evening while the sun disappeared behind the island in the sea.

Humbled and filled with gratitude, I blinked back tears that wanted to escape. Then I looked over at Dr. P who was watching Denise admire the ocean. I thought, *If everyone could witness such beauty and experience such compassion, surely there would not be so much suffering.*

"It is a magnificent display of God's beauty," Denise said, narrating the last of the golden hues that eventually blended into the blue-gray path to darkness.

"I could sit here forever and look out at this splendor," I sighed.

Contemplating what life would be like here, I stated aloud my feelings, "What a marvelous place this would be to sit and write." My thoughts breathed out of my mouth and into the dream I was surely creating.

I saw Dr. P watch me with a smile on his face and took a chance. "Want company?" I asked playfully. "I could stay here instead of going to Big Island for the summer."

"I leave for Iran in a few days, but if you want to come back next month, that may be possible," he responded.

A quick snap of my head brought my eyes right to his to see whether or not he was serious. My raised eyebrows asked before I did. "Do you mean I could come back?"

"Sure," he shot back with a shrug. "Why not?"

"That would be a dream come true," I whispered.

"Speaking of dreams coming true, what about that hot tub, Dr. P?" Denise chimed in. "Do you use it, or is it just for looks?"

"Oh, it's not for looks," he answered. "Would you like me to turn it on? And please, no more *doctor*, just call me P."

He walked over and switched on the pool lights that then glowed a bright, iridescent blue in the water as the hot tub bubbled through a spectrum of colors. The light display made us giggle like teenage girls.

"We don't have bathing suits," I said and looked at P inquisitively.

"Well, then," Denise said, "I guess we'll be going in our birthday suits. I do it all the time at home. This is Hawaii," she laughed.

P laughed as he walked off. "I'll grab some towels." Denise quickly undressed and walked over to the hot tub easing her way in. I followed right behind.

"Too hot?" I asked her.

"No, it's perfect," she cooed.

After a few minutes, P reappeared holding a few towels. Setting them down on the chaise, he slowly undressed and walked over to join us. With the first step in, his face scrunched up.

"That's quite warm." He took his time easing his way in, the whole while his face showing discomfort.

"Are you okay?" I asked, concerned.

"I had a little procedure done a few weeks ago," he said. "It's still a little sensitive. I probably shouldn't be in the water yet, so I won't stay in for too long." He spoke softly, under his breath, as if not wanting his words to be heard.

My heart felt a twinge of empathy. I picked up the concern in his barely audible words. I wondered what kind of procedure but didn't dare ask. I didn't want to impose on his privacy, but concern grew for him.

"I know you are a doctor and probably don't care for the way I do things," I said, "but like I told you, I've been healing with alternative modalities. Essential oils have helped me tremendously. If you are open to it, I would love to put some frankincense on the site where you had your procedure done. There are many health benefits to frankincense. It's an anti-inflammatory, for one, and some studies have shown it even helps with cancer."

Not thinking of his own expertise, I was eager to share my knowledge of another way to heal.

"Thank you, but I'll be fine," he said looking up into the night sky.

The three of us sat in silence for the next little bit, each of us taking in the brilliance of the milky way above. I wanted someone to pinch me to know if it was real, but at the same time, I wanted to live inside that dream forever.

~

A few hours later, were driving back to our condo when Denise looked over at me with a suspicious smile on her face. "I could see you staying here with P," she said. I looked over at her and smiled. I felt the same way.

"I mean it," she went on. "I could see you here helping each other with your healing. And I don't mean for just a week or two either."

"Yeah, right," I said. "Me? Here? With Dr. P? As much as I would love to, I don't think that is something P would be open to. I don't think he's open to hearing about energy healing or chakras and essential oils." I laughed at the picture in my mind. "I would love to come back before the summer is over and sit there and write my book. AND, maybe, just maybe, he would let me help around the house and cook him some healthy meals." My mind began to picture it, staying at P's, cooking in the big kitchen, sharing healthy meals with him, swimming in the pool, and listening to music.

The rest of that evening was spent writing in my journal and working on a new chapter in my book. Denise left to take a midnight stroll near the beach leaving me to my thoughts.

The week went by like a flash of lightning. During lunch on the final day of the conference, I asked my new friend, Kate, about areas to stay and places to explore on the island.

"Denise and I left our last two days unaccounted for," I explained to Kate. "We wanted to leave room for Spirit to bring some Maui magic into our lives. Do you have any recommendations from places to stay and things to do?"

"Hey, sorry," Denise cut in, pulling out the chair next to me. "I met a lady on the beach who has a condo that she's renting. She gave me her business card and said to call her by 3:00 pm if we want it, or we could use Airbnb or get a hotel."

"Well," I thought aloud, "in all honesty, I would love to ask P if we could stay there, but I don't want to impose. Can you imagine our last two nights there?" I squealed at the thought.

"Yes!" Denise agreed. "I could imagine that! Let's wait and see how the day unfolds."

Lunch with Kate slipped by quickly as did the afternoon classes. The conference came to an end and many of us exchanged numbers with several new friends. After the goodbyes were done, Denise and I found ourselves standing outside in the parking lot with no particular destination or a place to stay.

"Let's check out the rental the woman at the beach told you about," I suggested. In my heart, I was still hoping P would call and invite us, but I was losing hope.

When we arrived at the condo, there was loud music blaring from inside. Shoes were set outside the door and the windows were wide open. We called out, but no one answered. We knocked on the door, but no one came. Thinking the people may have gone for a stroll down the beach, we sat on the oceanfront lounge chairs and waited for someone to return.

We waited a good 30 minutes, and then we decided we should leave and find another option for the night.

"We need to find a place to stay," I laughed. "It's getting late. I was hoping P would call and invite us to stay there, but I guess he's busy tonight."

"Don't give up quite yet, Gail Lynn," said Denise. "Let's find some food and see where Spirit leads us." I let out a sigh of defeat. "Don't give up so easily," she repeated. "We'll find the perfect place. Besides, I imagined us there, too. Maybe he's still at work and will call soon."

"Let's go grab some food and head to the beach to watch the sunset," I said. "You're right. Spirit will lead us."

We got in the car and drove to a local market. We purchased two salads, a bottle of wine, and a wine opener. As we drove to find a beach, I tried to picture in my mind where P was at that moment when I was startled by the sound of my phone chirping. Looking at my phone, I saw his name.

"Oh my gosh, Denise!" I was shocked. "It's Dr. P! I was just picturing him in my mind." I held up the phone for her to see.

"Well, answer it, silly!"

"Aloha, Dr. P," I said. "How are you?"

"Good morning," his greeting made me smile. "I'm well, thank you. How was your day?"

"It was a good day, but sad saying goodbye to so many new friends. We just checked out of our condo, and we're heading to look for another place to stay."

"Oh, you don't have a place to stay?" he asked. "It's getting late. It may be hard for you ladies to find a place now. It's a busy time on Maui. Do you have somewhere in mind?"

"Denise got a recommendation for a condo unit," I explained. "The lady wasn't home when we got there, so now we're waiting to see if she comes back."

"Well, I have plenty of room here," he offered. "If you and Denise would like, you can stay here. You can each have your own room. Well, you may have to share with the kitties, but you are welcome to come if you'd like."

I slapped Denise on the leg in dumbfounded delight. "Are you sure you wouldn't mind having us?" I asked. "I mean, I would *love* to stay there. Let me check with Denise." She had pulled the car over and was smirking and nodding her head, wide-eyed and giggling like I was. "Dr. P invited us to stay at his house if we want," I told her as if she didn't know.

"Oh, how sweet," she exclaimed loudly. "You tell Dr. P we would *love* to take him up on his offer."

"I guess you'll have us as houseguests for the next two nights," I told him. "We'll stop at the store for some things on our way and be up in about an hour."

We giggled and clapped when I hung up the phone to celebrate what felt like Maui magic.

"See, Gail Lynn," she teased. "I told you not to give up. I've been picturing us up there at his beautiful house all day." We had both pictured it in our own ways and it had come to fruition.

I heard the voice of God, *Where two or more are gathered, there I am.*

"Thank you, thank you, thank you, God!" My heart was happy.

~

The next two days could not have been more perfect. While P was at work, Denise and I sat by the pool, walked in the gardens, hiked up the mountain to the Buddha garden, and sat in meditation. Each day when he returned from work, we retold our adventures of the day and how we had plenty to explore there on the property.

"We didn't want to go anywhere else," I told him, laughing. We were like a couple of silly schoolgirls dancing around the house while we cleaned up the kitchen to prepare dinner one night. "I feel like Cinderella," I said.

Our last night there, Denise and I wanted to cook up something special, but P wanted to go out.

"I was thinking pizza," he suggested. "There's a great little place not far from here. Would you like to take a ride in the Corvette?"

"Yes!" I shouted, excited to ride in the beautiful silver bullet that I had been admiring.

He looked at Denise. "Sorry," he apologized. "There's only room for one passenger. If you don't mind driving your car, I'll treat you to dinner." He smiled at me and melted my heart.

He asked if I minded riding with the top down, which of course I most certainly did not, especially with the evening sky as beautiful as it was. I wanted to ride with the wind whipping through my hair.

Within minutes we were flying down the West Maui mountain, Denise trailing behind us. The Corvette purred like a baby as P took up speed and raced around corners. Slowing down for the speed bumps, he looked over at me with a wide grin on his face.

When we turned onto the main highway, he shifted through the gears quickly, and I watched the humble doctor's adventurous spirit ignite. Racing down the highway made him happy. The speedometer hit 90 mph within seconds and his ear to ear smile made me laugh. He lit up like a little boy with a new toy.

At the pizza shop, dinner went by quickly. We each ordered a slice of pizza and a soda. P introduced us to the owner who offered us shaved ice and vanilla ice cream for dessert.

"You must try this," P insisted. "It's amazing. Mango and lime taste really good." We took his suggestion and enjoyed our dessert while seated at one of the sidewalk tables.

The whole evening sped by. Soon we were headed back home, the ride back even more thrilling as he pushed the speedometer to 100 mph. Within minutes we pulled up to the gate at the front of his property then stopped. Waiting for Denise to catch up, we sat looking at each other laughing until he reached over and brushed a strand of hair back away from my eyes. For a moment, I held my breath, waiting to see what he would do next.

Headlights caught our attention and the moment was lost. P opened the gate, revved up the engine, sped up to the top of the driveway, pulled in under the cover of the roof, and turned to me with a smile. I couldn't help being mesmerized by his charm.

"That was quite an adventure!" I laughed.

Denise walked over and offered to help put the cover back on while I floated on cloud nine. Watching the two of them again felt familiar. Once the Corvette was covered, I announced that I was going to get my bathing suit on and grab some towels.

"I'll meet you guys at the pool," I said. It was our last night there, and I wanted it to be special.

"Good, good," P said as he went inside followed by Denise. "I'll turn the hot tub on, and I'll grab some wine and the glasses."

It was an exceptionally warm evening. The milky way spread its beauty above us. I jumped in the pool, while Denise poured three glasses of Sauvignon Blanc and set them beside the hot tub. P turned on the heater and jets for the hot tub. It wasn't more than ten minutes when P stood up from the patio sofa and went to feel the temperature in the hot tub.

"It's ready whenever you are." He began to undress, placing all of his clothes on the back of the chairs. His tall lean body looked delectable. His sun-kissed torso changed shades of coloring where the waistline of his pants would have begun. I turned away blushing when he caught me staring. He simply smiled noticing my modesty at the sight of his naked body.

"It's too cold in New York to walk around naked all the time," I joked. "I'm not used to this. If my kids found out, they would think I've gone mad, and the neighbors would be aghast."

"Come on, Gail," Denise laughed. "Nudity is natural. When in Maui, do like the Maui-ans." She undressed and made her way into the hot tub as well. I wanted to make another joke about being the new *Three's Company,* but instead, I just hopped out of the pool, stripped off my bikini, and slid into the hot tub next to P. My heart fluttered beside him.

"Mmm, this is heaven," I purred. "Thank you, P for a lovely two days. I can't tell you how much it has meant to me, all that you've done. From the consultation about the

Lyme disease and writing an excuse for my employer to the dinners and sunsets and then inviting Denise and me to stay here in all of this. Inviting us to be your guests here in your lovely home is above and beyond what most people ever do. Most Americans don't even talk to strangers, let alone invite them for dinner."

Pausing, trying to find the right words, nothing seemed good enough. "I want you to know how much I appreciate you. You have made a difference in my life. You are my Earth angel."

I tried to refrain from getting too emotional, but my heart was on a roller coaster of emotions. I had this appreciation for P, a caring, a sense of love that I could not explain. The compassion that he had shown me has felt like a comforting embrace. Joy, love, kindness, these feelings were pushing my heart to expand greater than I had ever experienced.

As tears slid down my cheeks, I slid down underneath the water, hiding the emotions my heart couldn't help but reveal. When I came back up for air, tiny bubbles splashed water droplets onto my face blending with the salty tears. The thought of leaving in the morning made me melancholy. I didn't understand the feelings I was developing for P. It couldn't be love. Love doesn't happen that fast. Right? Or does it? I said a little prayer. *God, show me.* I looked over at P with a sense of admiration. He turned and looked at me, our eyes greeting each other with a tender smile as my heart connected to his.

"You're welcome," he said.

Denise sat with her head back watching the starry sky. "I am in awe of God's beauty," she said. Your place is magical, P. Thank you for inviting us to be your guests."

P smiled and nodded his head to Denise while, under the water, I felt his foot slide next to mine. His leg followed and rested up against my leg. Smiling, we looked up at the stars and he pointed out the Big Dipper right as a shooting star streaked across the evening sky.

"Make a wish you two," I squealed, laughing with excitement. I closed my eyes tightly and thought about my own wish.

"I'll call you next month when I get back from Iran," P said softly. "If you want to come back to write, you're welcome here with me."

My heart felt as if it was exploding out of my chest. If a heart could truly be cracked open, then that's what happened to mine. *Who is this man and where did he come from?* I asked myself again and again. Speaking to the angels, I asked over and over. *What is this magical experience? Is this all real?*

It was shortly after midnight when Denise and I finally went to bed. I fell asleep talking to God about these mystical experiences I was having.

~

The next morning, I woke up fully engulfed with good ole Mr. Fear Miser. I didn't want to get out of bed. I didn't want to gather my things and put them in the car. I didn't want to say goodbye to P. I was afraid I would never see him again. I laid in bed arguing with my thoughts, with God. *I know how this works. You bring this good into my life, tease me, then take it away.* Then Denise walked in. Her chipper self. She didn't know about all those people I cared about who had left me. I hid under the covers.

The conversations that I had in my head were endless. I talked with God, angels, the Fear, and even the little girl inside me. You know we all have that little child within that still seeks approval, seeks love. It's THAT which causes us to act the way we do. We're afraid we'll never find that... or lose it when it does fall into our lap... like now.

P will end up leaving me just like everyone else does, the little girl within bellowed out.

Then I begged God, *Don't let him forget about me. God, I think he's sad and alone just like me. We could be*

197

good for each other. I would take good care of him and help him find joy again.

Then Denise interrupted my thoughts. "Come on, Gail Lynn, we've got another adventure that begins today. Maui was good for you, now let Big Island give you some loving too!" I could hear her rustling with things.

I pulled back the covers and saw her holding up the outfit I had laid out the night before. "This is cute," she said. "Come on, get yourself together, and say goodbye to Dr. P and his kitties. You'll be back. Stop worrying."

Pouting, I got dressed, gathered my things, and went out to the lanai where Denise was already waiting. P's kitties, Cleo and Boy, came up to me and began rubbing their soft coats on my leg, purring, and meowing for attention.

"They see the suitcases and know you're leaving. They get mad whenever I leave. I see they have taken a fancy to you and are mad you're leaving too," P chuckled.

"I hope to see them again," I said. "I hope it works out to come back next month. Thank you for everything, P." I went over to him and wrapped my arms around his waist.

He pulled me in tighter. "You're welcome. I'll be in touch when I return." He leaned down and brushed my lips with a quick, gentle kiss. I stared up into his eyes. I knew those eyes. We had done this before, I just knew it.

The sound of Denise dragging her suitcase broke up our embrace. She came over to us, thanked him, and hugged him. "Let's go, Gail Lynn," she said. "You'll see Dr. P next month, so don't get all gushy," she chided. She knew me well.

I hugged P again and quickly got in the car.

We headed to the airport to catch our flight to the Big Island where we would meet up with Denise's sister, Wendy. We rode in silence to the airport, both of us enjoying the beauty of Maui's coastline.

"Don't worry, Gail Lynn," she reassured me. "He'll call. He'll invite you back. I could see it in his eyes. He

198

wants you there with him. I think you've left an impression on him as well."

I looked at her and smiled. "He's given so much to me Denise. I've never felt this before. Unconditionally, he has helped me with my job, he has given me compassion and cared about me, my health, my feelings. He's a gift the Universe, God, my angels brought into my life. I don't want to let go."

As the plane took off into the clouds, my mind swirled right along with the wisps of white that I stared at through the window. My body felt good. I had no symptom flare-ups. I forgot all about sickness and instead focused on the present moment, on the beauty of Maui, on what I had learned from the writer's workshop, and on the good feelings I had for P.

Each day in Maui was healing as I ate the local fruits and vegetables, played in the ocean, and laid in the hot sand. I knew all of it was healing my body, but it was also healing my heart and soul. I was sure of it. Part of me wanted to know which factors held the magic. Was it the writing? Was it the superfoods? The ocean? Or was it the compassion from P?

I journaled for most of the flight then opened my laptop and wrote more in my manuscript of my healing journey. I made a note to research the benefits of ocean water, sand, volcanic waters, sunshine, laughter, dancing, and chanting. Then I made one final note to remind myself to look up the power of love to heal. Maybe that was why God had put P and me together, to love and to heal. I closed up my laptop as the pilot said we were landing.

~11~

Interview At Heaven's Gate

Stepping off the plane on Big Island Hawaii, I was filled with mixed emotions. I was ecstatic about meeting Dr. P and was eager to tell Wendy the whole magical story, but I was also sad having to leave him and Maui behind.

Walking with Denise down the long corridor into the airport, I could feel energy beginning to build again. As soon as we saw Wendy, both she and Denise squealed with delight. Then Wendy turned and looked at me. "Come here, Gail Lynn, and give me a hug!"

Her warm embrace felt comforting, like a mother's. Then she pulled back, held onto my shoulders, and looked me straight in the eye. "I hear you have a spark in your heart," she said. "Is this man making you forget Bryce? How have you been feeling?"

I glanced over at Denise who looked like a cat caught with a mouse in her mouth. I raised my eyebrows at her in question. "Well..." I began my own version of the story that she had already heard second-hand from Denise. Part of me wanted to hear it again, though, so I began.

"First, there were all those problems I had with the school. They were demanding a doctor excuse and then threatened to fire me because I didn't have one. Well, then I got seated on my flight in Buffalo and I sat there wondering if I had made the right decision to leave school and take the risk of losing my job. I was in tears when the pilot called my name to get off the airplane because of some technical difficulty! I was really scared at that point! AND, the guy sitting next to me, he had to get off the plane too! I started talking to him about using alternative healing and going to a writer's conference and about trying to overcome the Lyme disease and then I mentioned Wayne Dyer – then guess what happened! He told me he is a doctor, Wendy!"

I was beside myself excited as I kept adding the details. "AND! Not only is he a doctor, BUT he was Wayne Dyer's doctor, Wendy! We got rerouted together for the eighteen hours to Maui. He conferenced with me the whole way about Lyme disease and then sent in a doctor's note to the school the next day. Then, Wendy, it gets even better, he invited us to dinner, then invited us to be his houseguests for our last two nights in Maui. I think I've died and gone to heaven. He's so kind and generous. He's tall and handsome and wise. I love talking with him. He's like a storage house full of information."

I kept babbling about the magical experiences I had in Maui when Wendy chimed in. "And look at you now, Gail Lynn! You look beautiful, you look healthy! It all sounds wonderful. Your healing journey has started out pretty amazing, I'd say. And now Big Island is going to take over and continue to love you up and bring you healing."

~

Later that evening, Wendy and I talked about making appointments with various energy healers. She told me about a sound healing event, a dance therapy at a local yoga center, and a workshop with a shaman. Before turning in for the night, we made plans to begin the next morning at the local market to gather some of the nutrient-dense local fruits and items I needed for my morning smoothies.

"We should turn in early and get a good night's sleep so that tomorrow we have lots of energy to explore the island," Wendy stated. "Perhaps you should call some of the people you met when you were here in April and set up some adventures with them."

In the morning, we decided to head to the local farmer's market. I bought papayas, avocados, watermelon, pineapple, and a new fruit I had never heard of called soursop. I didn't feel much like exploring, so we headed back home. As Wendy suggested, I called some friends that I had met back in April. I invited them over for an evening potluck so we could make plans for days of exploring.

As people arrived, Wendy made cocktails while Denise and I spread out the delicious food being brought in. We sat around the table and played with oracle cards while my friend Scott sifted through music. We laughed and caught up on what had happened since I was there in April.

Explaining to my Hawaii friends about the Lyme disease and the anxiety with the school situation I left behind, I told them about my plan for summer and alternative healing. That's when Scott pulled out a zip lock baggie and asked if I wanted a little smoke to ease my stress.

I wasn't exactly sure what it was, but I knew it wasn't tobacco. "Eek," I hesitated. "I'm a teacher, I don't think it's a good idea. Besides, I only put healthy stuff in my body. I haven't used drugs of any kind in years."

"This is medicinal marijuana," Scott replied. "People use it for all sorts of health issues. It helps ease any stress or anxiety and it's used for pain management. Maybe it will help you with the Lyme disease. You mentioned not being able to focus after the stroke you had, this could help that, too. Really, a lot of people use it to help ease their symptoms."

"I don't know," I said shaking my head. "Besides, I don't know how to smoke those things."

Scott took out a rolled cigarette-looking thing and lit it up. He took a puff then handed it to me. "See? It's no different than smoking a cigarette. You can't even tell this is weed," he laughed. "Come on, you'll feel better. Let all that stress go. You're on the island now, relax."

I reached over and took it, put it to my mouth, and wondered if it would really help. I took a puff, inhaled a little, then blew it out. It didn't hurt. I didn't feel anything, actually, so I did it again then handed it back to him, sat back in my chair, and listened to Wendy and Denise. They were looking through the music for a different CD to play. Scott handed me the rolled cigarette-like thing again and I took another puff. I began to feel more relaxed, so I took another puff then handed it to Scott.

"You're right!" I told him. "This is helping. But why is my mouth so dry?" I took a sip of wine.

"Take a drink of water," he said. "You'll be okay."

I looked back over at Wendy now sitting at the dining room table talking to Denise, and an odd feeling came over me. I felt a pinch in my chest and then a tightening so much that I had to hold my breath for a moment. My heart was racing. I felt lightheaded as the voices of Denise and Wendy echoed in my head. I stared at Wendy and tried to make sense of what she was saying.

"Wa-wa-wa… wa-wa…" I didn't understand what they were saying. But then words floated above her head in thought bubbles as she spoke. "Wa-wa-wa-wa-wa."

Then Denise had a thought bubble above her head. I could see her thoughts formulating in her mind before she spoke them aloud. It was very odd.

Then just as quickly as they had begun, the thought bubbles changed into an old black and white filmstrip. Moving backward in time, the film showed periods in my life, starting with my last day in New York. I had just finished working with my lawyer to complete a Last Will and Testament the day before I left for Hawaii. I placed it on the kitchen counter where it could easily be found.

That's interesting. Why did I do that? I thought.

In case you wanted to leave, I heard a voice respond.

The next frame of the filmstrip showed me standing outside my daughter's bedroom door. Sara was in her room, singing. She was sad, angry, and expressing emotions through the lyrics. She was mad at me, hurt. I suddenly realized I had failed her. I had let her down. My heart sunk in despair.

When that vision disappeared, another event appeared in the filmstrip, this time of my son, Josh. He was lying in bed after his accident. He was sad and angry and felt like giving up on life. Then I saw him as a child, and I was the one who was sad and angry and yelling at him. My heart hurt seeing this. Tears sprung from my eyes as I clutched my chest, witnessing myself get angry with my son.

The next vision came in just as quickly. There was James, my firstborn. He was a toddler, crying, screaming for me as I left him at a daycare. I had let him down.

Distraught with these scenes, my heart ached terribly for my children. They deserved better. I cried out to them in my mind. *I'm sorry, I'm so very sorry.* But they didn't hear. They were miles away.

Next came a scene with my ex-husband. He was standing beside our bed talking with me while our three children were upstairs watching television. I saw in his face that I'd let him down, too. I had just asked for a divorce.

I saw quick flashes of other times where I had made wrong choices, let others down, or brought sadness to someone in my life. I could feel all of the times where I had failed or caused someone pain. I was disgusted with myself. Instantly, I knew I was dying. This was my life review. I was ready.

I tried to get Wendy's attention.

"Wendy, I don't...feel so well," I muttered. "I need to go lie down." I heard myself say these words, yet I couldn't remember my mouth moving to form them. I was unsure if I had thought or spoke them. I looked at Wendy, and everything began to move in slow motion. The sofa was maybe 20 feet away.

We need to get to the sofa, I told myself.
Who is "we"? I asked myself. *Who am I?*

~

A deep sorrow filled me. Sliding down off of the stool, I took a step towards the sofa. With great remorse, I spoke to those memories.

I'm sorry, I said.

Everything went dark. Like an evening without stars or moonlight, lost in the cosmos of outer space, I felt myself lifting in flight, up into another realm.

When I opened my eyes, it was dark still, yet there was a golden hue of color radiating out, comforting me. A symphony of music welcomed me. The golden light expanded and at first, I thought I was in a grand ballroom. I felt joy and an inner sense of peace. I felt loved, great love. The concerto, the masterpiece of life, unfolded before me as I entered this state of what felt like coming home. A bright light illuminated the silhouettes of several people, all standing with their backs to me.

Why do they have their backs to me? I wondered.

Confused by this image, I turned my head and noticed white puffy clouds around my midsection. Oddly, I could put my hand through them. I could see my body stretched through the clouds, elongated down through the atmosphere to what appeared to be the Earth. My feet were stuck there. Like my sons Stretch Armstrong toy, my body extended from the place on Earth where my feet had been planted to this place above the clouds in the cosmos, the multi-verse, the unknown.

Am I dead? I wondered. Maybe this was heaven. *Is this what it feels like to die?*

I floated in space feeling a great love surround me. My heart felt full of awe and wonder. I felt loved. I wanted more. I tried to reach up and pull myself more fully into this other place, but I could go no further.

That's when the angel appeared.

Two beings rode up in an ancient chariot. One held the reins and the other held what appeared to be a scroll. They looked like men from long ago, perhaps Egyptian, or Roman. Stopping a short distance away, the one who held the scroll moved closer. He was dressed in white garbs with golden cords draped across his shoulder. Feathery wings appeared in form behind him and then quickly disappeared. He radiated energy in a light that held me in suspense until he drew apart his hands, top to bottom, unrolling the scroll. I stood there in amazement as I read it.

Angel of Free Will.

The rest of the scroll was unreadable, written in a print I could not understand. It felt familiar, though, as if I should know, as if I had used the words before. I looked at the angel who held the scroll and waited for him to speak. I could hear his thoughts.

You choose.

I understood. *This is how telepathy works,* I thought back to him.

It was my choice if I wanted to stay in heaven or return down to Earth. I thought another answer back to him.

I want to go further up.

Again, I leaned forward and tried to reach my arms up to pull myself higher into this heavenly realm. Yes, it was beautiful, it was loving and kind. It was what everyone on Earth searched for. As much as I tried to pull myself up though, I could not.

Your children need you, I heard.

The people still had their backs to me. I could not see who spoke, or if perhaps it was God's voice. I looked back at the angel who was staring at me, waiting.

Then a series of pictures flashed through my mind. One by one, I saw each of my children engaged in life, busy as ever. My heart felt heavy.

They will be okay, I told the angel in my thoughts.

Then I looked into the future and saw my own funeral. My heart ached even more. I did not want to see the suffering that I would cause. I wanted to go higher. I wanted to fully enter the gates of this heaven and be encompassed by the love that was emanating out towards me. I kept reaching up, but I couldn't move. Then I saw my children again. They were busy, confused, struggling through life.

Your children need you, the voice said again.

At the brink of fully accepting heaven as my new home, I suddenly became aware of the erroneous knowledge that I had taught my children. For many of their childhood years, their father and I had brought them to church where they learned *mistakes* about who and what God and heaven really was. They were taught rules, not universal truths of the World, but truths of men who wanted control.

Heaven wasn't a place above the clouds, it was a state of being, it was this consciousness. Heaven, as Jesus taught, was within. The kingdom of God was within. It was this *feeling* of being fully aligned with universal, *unconditional* love. That was the true experience of heaven. This place, this space in the cosmos, it was a continuation of that which is below.

As above, so below, the angel thought to me.

Then I saw my own life. Where I had a negative thought in my mind (as above), it came to be in my life (so below). The fears I thought about, I brought in through focusing on them. *The only thing to fear is fear itself,* the angel thought to me.

I get it.

Hanging my head in disappointment, I was now battling my inner demons. The negative experiences in our lives are our own doing. I caused it all by fearing the worst. I was ashamed of myself.

I had caused the break-up with Bryce because I feared he would leave me. I didn't feel like I was lovable.

The angel drew nearer and spoke softly in thought. *Love the Lord your God with all your mind, with all your heart, with all your soul. You! Love yourself. Forgive as you have been forgiven.*

I wanted to go into the form of energy that knew not the earthly burdens that weighed us down. This, the high vibration where we experienced Oneness and wholeness and love from all who had gone before us, is what I've been seeking. *I get it,* I thought out again to the angel. *I need to return.*

I need to teach my children, my sister, and my brothers. When we remove the low vibrations from our daily life, we will begin to walk and enter the kingdom of heaven, the place of true consciousness. Sickness enters when our vibration is low. When we are in the high vibration of love, sickness can't enter, unless we owe a karmic debt.

Begin to know thyself better, my inner voice stated.

You are love. You are the gift!

~

I felt a struggle between my lower self, the child within, the girl named Gail, and the higher aspect of me, my higher consciousness. The whole time I was having this inner dialogue between the different parts of me, my angel stood watching, waiting. The struggle was real. I had searched my whole life to feel this love yet knowing now that I had taught my children all wrong, I had to go back to Earth. I had to go back and teach my family differently. I had to correct my mistakes. This was my chance to make things right with my children.

You choose, said the angel once more.

I turned and looked at the being who stared at me.

Yes, I will return, I thought telepathically back to the angel.

As soon as I said that, another man appeared. He was tall and handsome with bare feet, long hair, and a robe of purest white.

Jesus? I whispered.

His deep-set eyes held fast onto mine. He extended two fingers out and touched me where my shoulder met my arm. Without moving his lips, he spoke.

I love you. Go heal, go teach.

And with that, I fell back down through the dark sky, through the cloud back where I came from.

~12~

The Return

When I opened my eyes, my body was on a table in an emergency room, surrounded by doctors and nurses. The one holding the paddles, like two yellow suns side by side above my chest, yelled out, "Clear!"

The nurse brought the paddles to my chest. I watched as my lungs filled with air as everyone looked on at the monitors. It was confusing and intriguing all at the same time as I hovered in the corner aware that I was watching my*self* on a table surrounded by doctors.

I became blinded by a bright light after that and felt my body floating again until a few minutes had passed. I heard familiar voices, and then there was a pungent smell. I tried turning away from the smell, but I couldn't move. I tried again and heard another familiar voice. I was no longer the observer. I was back in my body, coughing and pushing at something that was crowding my face.

Twisting and writhing to get away from the awful smell, I became aware that I was bound by something that held me down. I noticed I was losing that feeling of love that I had experienced moments earlier. I reached out and grabbed the hand of Jesus. Then a more fragrant smell came closer. It was a beautiful scent that made me feel connected once again to that love. I tried opening my eyes to see him again, but the light hurt. As I lifted my hand to block the glare and slowly open my eyes, I saw Jesus standing before me. He was holding a Hawaiian Plumeria flower.

Jesus, I whispered. I closed my eyes and shook the fogginess out of my head.

Slowly, I opened them again and there was Scott standing in front of me, wide-eyed, fanning a plumeria in front of my nose.

I began crying as I looked up at Scott. "You're Jesus?" I asked.

Cradled like a baby in Wendy's arms, I wept as she rocked me back and forth. "Thank you, Jesus!" she sang out. "Thank you, thank you!"

She stopped to gaze into my eyes and suddenly spoke. "Gail Lynn," she scolded me sternly. "You had us all scared to death! Miss Denise here has tried calling 911 three times now and hasn't been able to get through. Scott has been waving that damn flower in front of your nose, and I've been praying to God that you return to us!"

She pulled me in closer and rocked as we both cried.

I was confused and tired. Wendy pulled back and looked down at me, and I told her what had happened.

"I saw Jesus," I whispered. Then I looked up at Scott who was still standing over me. "It was you. You were Jesus. You touched me, didn't you?" He nodded yes.

"I wanted to stay," I said and turned to look at Wendy. "I wanted to be with him. I felt so loved. I'm sorry, I did not want to come back. My feet were stuck to the Earth and I couldn't go any further. I kept reaching and trying to pull myself up, but an angel appeared and unrolled a scroll for me to read. He said I had a choice. That's what free will means, that we have a choice. Every day we have free will. The angel told me that my kids needed me. I didn't believe the angel, but then I saw my kids here. I knew I had to come back and teach them about love and healing. Heaven is just a state of mind. We create our own heaven or hell."

Wendy rocked me some more. "You are loved right here, Gail Lynn," she said. "We all love you."

"I love you too, Gail Lynn," Denise planted a kiss on my forehead. "You gave me quite the scare."

Scott reached down and held my hand. "You have many who love you, Gail."

Too tired to talk further, I smiled and closed my eyes.

Wendy began to give orders for people to bring food over, for Denise to start some hot water for tea, and for Scott to go to the washroom and get a wet washcloth for my head to keep me awake.

When I looked up at Wendy, I could still see the worry in her face. "I'm not going anywhere," I assured her. "Don't worry. I'm back. I have to teach people about the other side of life. Jesus gave me a gift. We get the gifts of prophecy and healing when we go into the light."

~

My death experience, seeing Jesus and meeting with the collective consciousness, was freeing. That night I had many dreams and visions, and those visions came to me more and more frequently afterward. That night I spoke to Jesus and the angels and the Divine Intelligence that permeates all around us.

There's no need to fear death anymore, I heard. *You know it is your thoughts and fears that bring on death. By your words, it is done. Your beliefs are changing. That is good. Keep searching.*

In the next few days, I had very little energy and slept more than usual. Denise and Wendy went off exploring while I stayed in to think, write, and reflect on life. I was suddenly seeing everything around me in brighter colors. The sounds of nature were more magical. Life seemed different. I could hear things, see things, feel things more clearly. Not just in the earthly realm, but in the spiritual realm as well.

There were things that I just KNEW. I didn't know what to make of it.

A few days later, Denise left to go back to New York for work, and I was left to my own thoughts again throughout the day as Wendy went off to work. After a few days of staying confined to the house and yard, she began to encourage me to get out and explore the Big Island.

"There is so much to see and do, Gail Lynn. Don't let that little experience you had trouble you. You've been awfully quiet. It's time for you to get out and explore. Take Laurie's car tomorrow and go sit at the warm ponds. That's the place Laurie took you when you were here in April."

So much was happening in my head I had no desire to go off on my own, not yet. I was processing so many feelings, memories, traumas. I was also thinking about my children and my inability to be a good mother for so many years. I needed to tell them I was sorry. I needed to ask for forgiveness.

The next morning, I awoke and noticed the calendar. It was July 3rd already. Time had flown by. I decided I would go explore that day, so after breakfast, Wendy packed me a bag of goodies and herself a lunch bag. She got out snorkel gear, a beach bag, and a water bottle. "Go have fun," she said, handing them to me.

While driving the winding roads and thinking about the warm ponds, my mind began to wander back to that initial visit. I remembered floating in the warm ponds with Laurie day after day and feeling a sense of peace and relief. I looked forward to just floating again. I wanted to clear my mind of everything that had happened. I knew I needed to prepare myself for teaching again. I needed to get stronger and I needed to talk with the angels again to learn how.

There were very few people at the warm ponds. I made my way down the path to the side where I could lay out my towel and bask in the full rays of the sun. I took in the clear blue sky and warm sunshine for an hour, warming my skin before entering the water. Ready to cool off, I grabbed the foam noodles and entered the warm pond at the back where it was warmer. As my body adjusted to the temperatures, I swam closer and closer to the break wall where the ocean water crashed up and over into the pond.

Within minutes I could feel the vitality in my body rising. I felt more limber and flexible and more energetic. I dove down under the water and swam a few feet until I could no longer hold my breath. I remember when I could swim the length of our pool underwater, but after the Lyme, oftentimes it hurt when I got into the water, and holding my breath for very long was a big task. I floated with one noodle under my head and another under my feet, closed my eyes, and drifted into meditation. I visualized the water of the warm ponds entering through my skin and communicating with the water and cells in my body. I pictured the atoms and molecules talking to each other. It was so easy, so natural like I could access deeper imagery inside of my mind. I heard a voice tell me to research it and saw the words float through my mind: *magnesium, potassium, calcium, phosphorus, sulfur, minerals, lava, volcanoes.*

Time passed quickly, and before I knew it, my stomach was crying out for food. I made my way back to my towel and pulled out the mango first. Opening the pocketknife, I slowly began cutting slices off and then bit into each piece savoring every bite. I laughed at the juices dripping down my arm. I felt like a kid, naïve with both the pocketknife and the mango. Next, I grabbed the avocado and sliced it in half. Using the blade, I swiped out the insides, stabbed at it, then carefully put one half in my mouth. I did the same with the other half then tossed the pit aside as I went to the water to rinse off my knife. Stomach satisfied, I shifted the towel to get more sun then sat and pulled out my journal.

As my eyes drifted to the sky and then to the people around the warm pond, I suddenly felt an uneasy feeling, as if I was being watched. Two fellas across the pond were seated on a bench engrossed in conversation and another guy up in the lifeguard station appeared occupied as well. Realizing I was the only woman here with these three men, I began to feel uncomfortable. I quickly packed up my things and headed to my car. As I walked up the path past the pavilion, one of the guys who had been watching me called out, "Leaving so soon?"

I waved politely and commented on something about making dinner for my family. It was an eerie feeling. *Had they been watching and talking about me?* I wondered.

As I neared the car, a monarch butterfly fluttered around my head. It made me think of Wayne Dyer, so I spoke to the butterfly. "Hello, Wayne."

The butterfly followed me as I walked to the back of the car and opened the trunk. It fluttered about as if trying to tell me something, so I began to talk to it and ask it questions.

"What's up, Wayne? Are you trying to tell me something?" Another monarch showed up. "Oh, hello!" I greeted it. "And who are you?" The two flitted about in front of me as if trying to get my attention. "Are you two trying to tell me something?"

I didn't *hear* anything, but a strong feeling of worry came over me. I panicked as a thought rushed through my mind that tomorrow was the Fourth of July. Then I remembered Wayne's story. When the monarch showed up for him, he knew it was his friend from the spirit world.

"Did someone cross over into the spirit world? Did something happen to one of my children?"

I asked aloud as if Wayne would answer me through the butterflies. I recalled how this holiday had been a difficult day in my family for the past few years and I began to panic.

First, I called Josh, but there was no answer. I texted.
Hey Josh, you okay? What are you doing?
Then I sent a text to James.
Hey honey. How's it going? I miss you.
Next, I tried calling Sara. No answer. I texted her.
Hey, how are you? Everything okay? Miss you.

Each of my three kids responded back within a few minutes. They were all doing well. Silly me. Nothing was wrong. I looked at the two butterflies still flitting about and felt silly, so I got in the car and drove back to Wendy's. She was already in the kitchen preparing salads for us when I walked in.

"How was your day?" she asked. "Explore any place new?

I told Wendy about my meditation at the warm ponds and how good it felt to just float effortlessly. We talked about the healing salts and the sulfur of the water and I shared with her my thoughts on researching the health benefits. I skipped over my experiences with the butterflies and the eerie feeling of being watched at the warm ponds. We put a movie on after dinner and went to bed right after.

The sound of my phone startled me out of deep sleep. I reached over to grab it off the nightstand and saw a text message from my daughter-in-law's mother back home in New York. She must have forgotten the six-hour time difference because it was quite early. I opened it anyway.

Debby died.

I sat up instantly, wiped the sleepiness from my eyes, and called her to hear the sad news of a loved one crossing over into the spirit world. Then I remembered the butterflies.

Death. What an interesting phenomenon. I found it hard to grieve this loss when I knew the beauty of what was on the other side. Debby was enveloped in love. I was happy for her. I knew people would not understand, so I said nothing more. The butterfly is such a beautiful metaphor for what happens at death. We become changed, not dead. *Our soul never dies*, I said to myself. *Why don't people understand that?*

I got out of bed to find Wendy. She was already getting ready for work and putting her makeup on. I went up behind her and wrapped my arms around her waist, resting my head on her back.

"A friend back in New York died sometime last night," I told her. "Everyone is sad, but Debby is free now." I thought about that for a moment. "I don't know whether to be happy or sad. I feel empty, but I also feel everything, all their feelings of sadness."

"I'm sorry for the loss in your family, Gail Lynn. You know love never dies," she said. "You know our soul goes on forever. If she's happy, that's all that matters. Let yourself feel whatever you want to feel. It's okay, sweetie."

I grabbed my journal from the nightstand and went to the lanai to write. Wendy came out a few minutes later with coffee for us both then sat down beside me.

"Some days I just feel numb," I told her. "I think about my experience of almost dying and meeting Jesus and I feel like I should be happy that I'm alive. I feel like I should go back to New York to be with the family during this loss. I was feeling mixed emotions. I didn't die, Debby did. How do I tell people that we get to choose life or death? We have free will."

"You're doing fine, Gail Lynn," she assured me. "Just take things one day at a time. I'll be home for lunch. I took the afternoon off so I could show you around a bit. Maybe you should consider moving here and teaching here. Hawaii needs teachers." Smiling, Wendy picked up her coffee mug and headed out the door. "Call me if you need to talk, otherwise I'll be home in the afternoon."

~

I began to think about the warm ponds and remembered that I wanted to look up the health benefits of mineral springs. I spent the morning researching. One website after another schooled me on the benefits of hot springs. I found articles and took notes on Balneotherapy that dated back to Rome, Greece, France, and the days of Jesus and Mary Magdalene at the Sea of Galilee. I read about the Greek physician Hippocrates who wrote on the healing powers of waters and using saline baths to cure ailments. I read about Cleopatra and other ancient Egyptians who used water therapy and how they often visited the Dead Sea to soak in the mineral-rich waters. I read about pharmaceutical companies and cosmetic factories that have established places near salty shores to take full advantage of the health benefits of locations near the sea.

Fascinated, I spent hours online reading essays, articles, and historical findings. From my notes, I began to make connections to my own health improvements beginning in April when I first started to sit in the warm ponds. When Wendy got home, I told her of my discoveries.

"How do people NOT know this stuff?" I was flabbergasted at the vast amount of information I had found in such a short time of researching.

"Well, Gail Lynn, not everyone wants to do the work," she said. "They are willing to pay the big bucks for doctors to tell them what to do. OR they don't know where to begin researching."

"Wendy, throughout history, bathing in mineral-rich waters was helpful in curing many ailments. The Romans were well known for Balneotherapy until the collapse of their empire around 540AD, at which time they abandoned the practice of therapeutic bathing. Over the years, the Roman Catholic Church began to discourage people from public watering places, citing a strict moral code. So, it was the Romans who began speaking out against it. Perhaps they didn't want people to know of this ancient mystery and wanted to keep the secrets of these health benefits to themselves in order to pursue personal gain. WOULD THEY DO THAT?" I was aghast at my findings.

"It's hard to say these days what people know and don't know," Wendy said. "I would hope the church isn't keeping important information from people."

"I swear, my body knew Hawaii had healing to offer me. That's why I felt so called here. And just think, the principal and administrators wanted to stop me. Guess what else, they are Roman Catholics. Is that a coincidence? Is it possible that they somehow *wanted* me to stay sick? Subconsciously?" The thought made me shiver.

I was disgusted and couldn't keep the scowl off my face. "You know, I taught my students about the water cycle and I shared a book with them by Dr. Masaru Emoto, *The Hidden Messages in Water*. In it, he shows water crystals that have been exposed to classical music and positive words. The water responded by vibrating into beautifully formed crystals that he photographed. Then he did the same experiment but exposed the water to offensive music and negative words, and the water vibrated into imperfect and ugly shapes. Do you know what it all means?" I asked her excitedly.

"I do not," Wendy laughed. "Please, tell me."

I laughed right along with her. I was so excited about my discovery. I told her how Spirit had led me to find this information to put it all together.

"It's like water has its own set of ears," I said. "It has intelligence. It listens and then responds in like manner. Whatever your words, music, sounds, and thoughts are, you will get it back. If they are loving, you'll get a loving response. If you put out words and feelings of love, peace, joy, and happiness around water, and since our body is over 75% water, then we can speak words *into* our own body of water! MY body! Your body! We can do self-healing by the power of our thoughts and words!"

I was over the top excited with my research and theories. I continued as she stared at me in wonder. "And the water of the warm ponds and the people in it who feel love and happiness and probably laugh as they jump in, their positivity enhances the mineral content even more! It helps people *if* they can begin to change their *own* emotions and thoughts to a positive vibration because like attracts like!"

Wendy and I met eyes and burst out laughing at my elation.

I continued as if concluding my speech. "I needed to be here for my healing journey. The mineral content of the warm ponds is exactly what my body was missing. It's why I felt so at peace and why my body began to feel good after I was here in April."

"If only your school could see you now!" Wendy cheered. "Look at the improvements that you've made in this short time. Between the magic of Maui and the Big Island, you have your health back!"

Each day forward, I made a conscious decision to go to the warm pond daily for a least an hour. I thought about the volcano Pele here that was constantly flowing, assisting us with life, and I closed my eyes and said a little prayer of thanksgiving to her. I imagined the warm pond providing minerals and sulfur to my body and reducing inflammation and gave thanks.

I thought about the flare-up of symptoms that had occurred each month and imagined what it would have been like these past four years if I had only had hot springs to bathe in. If I had only had this knowledge for the past four years. Maybe the pain would have disappeared immediately. I thought about the dead spirochetes of the Lyme that die off and the toxins that get trapped inside the body that need to escape. I wondered if the hot springs could be the answer to the pain for so many other people. I was eager to test my ideas out and wondered how else I could get rid of the toxins that were still in my body.

Day after day I went to the warm ponds to swim and meditate. I wrote and ate raw fruits and vegetables. Each day brought a new experience, a new lesson to learn, a fear to overcome, an opportunity to love, or to be of service.

One day I drove to the water filling station and came across a woman who was hitchhiking. Something came over me. Going against everything I was ever taught, I pulled over to the side of the road to see where she was going. She was thin, scraggly, had a bandana tied around her head, and was carrying a backpack that looked as if it weighed just as much as her, if not more. My heart went out to her. I wanted to help.

"Where you headed?" I asked.

"I need to get my water bottle filled. I need to get to a market for food." Her voice crackled as she breathed heavily. I motioned for her to get out of the hot sun and into the backseat. She grabbed her backpack and hopped in and immediately asked if I had any water. All I had was my own bottle, but she was sweaty and pale and looked sickly, so I offered it to her.

"I'm heading down to Uncle Robert's to grab a bite to eat," I said. "What's your name?"

"I'm Debra," she replied. "There's a church mission on the way. You can drop me off there if it's no bother."

In the rearview mirror, I could see that her cheekbones were protruding. "Would you like to join me for lunch? I'd like to treat you."

She was grateful, more than grateful. I bought her lunch and then loaded her up with apples, mangoes, and oranges before taking her to the mission. I completely forgot about my own mission to get the water bottles filled up for Wendy. Later that night when I shared with her about my day, I told her how that was one of the scariest things I had ever done, picking up a hitchhiker.

"That's how a lot of people get around here on the island," she told me. "People carpool and rideshare and do a lot of walking or hitchhiking. I hope you know enough not to pick up a man when you are by yourself though."

"Yes, Wendy," I laughed. "I really don't know what came over me. Spirit was telling me she needed help, so I had to. I ended up having a great conversation with her and it felt so right. Like Dr. P was my Earth angel, I can be that for others."

"That's what we do on the island, sweetie. We help each other out."

When the weekend rolled around, Wendy said that she wanted to show me some of the schools and different houses for sale. "I think you would love living here. Embracing a healthy way of life with healing events like the Five Rhythm Dance and yoga nearby is right up your alley. You can teach all you have learned about healing."

After a few hours of enjoying the beautiful sunny day with a meditative swim, we drove back towards the Puna district and then down to Uncle Robert's.

Wendy pointed out the window. "This is called the Red Road. You can feel the power of Pele here. Just look at those sharp edges on the old lava formations."

We continued down the road and enjoyed the beautiful vistas until we came to a large lawn that divided the road. There were many people, some with hula hoops, others doing yoga, and a few with drums. We circled around and then headed back the way we came. We had gone about a mile when we passed a hitchhiker.

"Wendy!" I shouted. "We have to stop!"

She slammed on the brakes and pulled over. "What? What's wrong?"

"That man is hitchhiking. We have to stop and help him," I said. The gray-haired man was now walking toward our car. I rolled down my window part way.

"I need a lift into Pahoa," he said. "Are you headed that way?"

Wendy and I exchanged a look then she asked him what he was going to do in Pahoa.

"I'm headed to the Natch to meet up with friends for dinner," he filled us in on the details of his day. "I live in that area but came here for morning yoga." He pointed back to the lawn we had just passed.

I looked over at Wendy with pleading eyes. I hated the idea of this old man having to walk all that way back into town. She smiled kindly and told the man to get in the back seat.

"I'm Jacob," he said. "Thank you for the lift. I could have walked it, but I've been in the sun all afternoon doing yoga. I'm happy to have a ride." He had long, lean arms and his face was tanned but thin with piercing eyes and a big smile.

We introduced ourselves then Wendy began a line of questions about what he does here on the island and how long he's been here. We learned that he was a world traveler and that he knew a lot of good spots on the island that Wendy didn't know about. He was 74 years old and honored us with an impressive demo of his powerful chanting voice.

When we pulled into the Island Naturals Market, he handed me his business card and told me to call him if I wanted a tour guide. He got out and thanked Wendy for the ride.

When Jacob was out of sight, she scrunched up her face and began scolding me. "Gail Lynn, don't ever shout like that at me while I'm driving!"

I looked at her, hesitated for just a moment, then burst out laughing.

"I'm sorry. I didn't mean to startle you while you were driving, but I am so amazed at how easily we can open our hearts to loving people and BAM, God puts people in our lives to help. It feels great to help and make a difference in someone's life."

~

Later that night, we talked about Jacob and his offer to show me around the island.

"I booked a flight for us to go to Oahu for the weekend!" Wendy exclaimed. "I thought you would like to visit Pearl Harbor memorial while you're here. But you should give Jacob a call and let him show you around the island when we get back."

"I'll see how it feels when we return," I told her.

On Friday, we boarded the island hopper to Oahu. Something was a little unsettling. When we landed, I immediately felt the charged energy of the island, much more chaotic than the laid-back feeling on Big Island. We went for

224

dinner and turned in early to prepare for the long day ahead of us.

Waking up the next day, I began to feel anxious and more unsettled about going to see Pearl Harbor. I couldn't explain it. There was just an uneasiness.

When we arrived, an immediate sense of sadness struck me. People weren't smiling. Men, women, and even children were walking around with their eyebrows furrowed with grimaces on their faces. Parents were hushing their children.

After going through the gate, our first stop was to watch a documentary. It was filmed in black and white and portrayed the events leading up to the attacks. I had a sick feeling as I became angry at the Japanese for the war, but as the documentary continued, I became angry at the Americans. By the end, I was angry at all the men involved because I could see that behind the war was unnecessary greed and control. I wanted to leave.

We were ushered out. Wendy wanted to tour the submarine. Something inside me was screaming at me not to go, but I didn't want to let her down. I felt sick. Visions started to come to me of bombs dropping. Wendy started to go down the stairs into the submarine. I began to follow her down, but panic stopped me. I quickly climbed back up and raced back across the bridge to find a bench to sit. I was restless, though.

Visions came flooding into my mind of myself, as a nurse, running across an open field. A bomb came, exploded nearby, and I fell to the ground. There weren't many people around, just a sailor. I knew him. He was my lover. In the vision, he ran to me and lifted me up, but I died there in his arms as he told me, "I love you, forever."

~

We visited a few other tourist attractions the next day and then flew out that night. Flying over the ocean back to

Big Island, I contemplated who that sailor was from the vision I had on Oahu. It felt like a past life that I wanted to know more about.

The next day before going off to work, Wendy reminded me to give Jacob a call.

"What do you have to lose?" she asked. "Keep exploring Big Island!"

I summoned up the courage and called him the following day. We set a time to meet at the Island Market in Pahoa for lunch. He seemed nice enough and told me about his travels to Thailand and Australia. We talked about religion and I was impressed with his knowledge.

"Why don't you join me this Sunday," he insisted. "First, I go to a service with the Christian Scientists, then head to a Synagogue, and then end the day chanting Hare Krishna and sharing a meal of soup and fresh vegetables at a local temple."

I accepted. I didn't know anything about any of those practices, and I was open to learning. All the beliefs around the world are quite similar and what *is* different doesn't matter. We are all learning. I didn't tell him I had a near-death experience or that I had died and met Jesus. I just wanted to take it all in.

After our lunch, he wanted to show me one of his favorite beach spots, and I accepted but drove myself there in case I needed to escape. It was a short drive to a cliff where we started walking. The path was steep. I was a little worried if I could make it, but I told my body it would be easy.

Water consciousness, I kept thinking to myself. *Our body listens to our words and thoughts.*

Trekking down the path was an adventure in itself, but once we got to the bottom and I picked my head up to look around, I noticed it was a nude beach.

I was uncomfortable but wanted to fit in, so after a few minutes of assessing the situation, I undressed and laid face down on my beach towel. Hawaii had taught me many new things about how to experience life differently and how to heal. Jacob undressed and began socializing right away. At first, I found it funny watching people greet one another hugging their naked bodies together, but then I took notice of how natural it looked. No one gawked or stared or made any sign of being uncomfortable. It was only me who laid there feeling out of sorts. Jacob came back, reached out his hand, and asked me to join him for a swim.

I took a deep breath and stood up. Walking to the edge of the water, he warned me of the strong current. He wasn't kidding. As the first wave met my knees, I stumbled and fell, getting tossed about like an inflatable toy. Grabbing hold of me, he pulled me up and wrapped an arm around me as I coughed and blew the water out of my nose.

"I'll hold onto you if you need," he laughed.

Odd as it was in my nakedness, I clung to him for dear life like a baby clinging to a parent. I didn't want to leave the waters. I wanted to be brave like the others and to swim on my own, but thankfully he held onto me so that the strong current didn't pull me out to sea.

When we got back to our towels, he sat and pulled a baseball cap out of his bag to cover his eyes from the bright sun.

"I'll meet you in dreamland," he said as he laid down for a nap. I pulled out a book to read. I forgot about being naked and just soaked up the sun and pleasure of the wind on my body. I chuckled at the thought of people back home gossiping if they got wind of this. Most east coast folks were so rigid. We're born naked, but somewhere along the way, we are taught that it is wrong or bad to be seen naked.

Jacob snoozed for about an hour before finally rising. When he did sit up, another gentleman from across the way noticed him and walked towards us. I stifled a laugh at the thought again of my friends back home. *If only they could see me now, sitting here watching these butt naked men chit chat.* I laughed.

The afternoon hours passed, and I got fidgety with the want to get home and write. I told Jacob I wanted to leave.

"What? Write?" he was shocked. "You're going to leave me and this beautiful beach to go write? Tell me about this story you're writing." He probed and probed and seemed fixated on knowing what I had written and how far I was into the story. I kept it brief and told him he'd have to wait until it was finished.

"Look around you," he said. "You are on the Big Island. Why not just enjoy your time exploring with me? Forget about the book. You can write when you go back to New York."

An odd feeling came over me. I stood and grabbed my flip-flops and backpack and told him we'd be in touch. I didn't have to explain myself or my desire to get home. I thanked him and waved goodbye, but he stood and stretched out his arms.

"What, no hug?" he asked, and as if it wasn't awkward enough, I went up to him, fully unclothed, and gave him an embrace. He squeezed tight and began to chant. I stood there for a moment and allowed the sounds to vibrate through my body. The sound of his voice was comforting.

"I don't know what *that* was," I said when we stood back and looked at each other, "but it was beautiful."

"Aramaic, love. It was sounds of healing for you."

I thanked him again and walked towards the path that led up the side of the cliff to my car.

When I finally arrived home and filled Wendy in about my day, she laughed and congratulated me on having new experiences. I told her about Jacob questioning my book and how it felt really strange that he kept pushing to know more about my writing.

"He was pushing me to spend time with him instead of working on my writing. It's like he was trying to distract me from my work."

"The island will take care of you, Gail Lynn," she reminded me. She calmed my fear by chalking him up to be a curious old man who enjoyed my company. "You're safe here."

The rest of the night was quiet. We chatted out on the lanai into the night, and then I listened to my favorite Wayne Dyer meditation under the stars. "I Am That I Am" lulled me into a deep meditative state and connected me with Wayne. I saw him smiling with one hand over his heart. I awoke and felt the peaceful warmth of the night. I thought about P and wondered if he would call. I thought about Jacob and his chanting. I contemplated calling him, but decided to wait, then went inside to unscramble my thoughts with some writing.

Dear Source...
I want to say thank you for everything. Please help me to know what to do next for my healing. Please help me to know what to do about Jacob. Please help me with writing my book.

~

The next day I decided to give Jacob a call. He invited me over for lunch and to meet his roommate. When I arrived, his friend was resting in bed. Jacob had just finished doing energy work on him to help relieve the pain from a shoulder injury.

"I didn't know you were an energy healer," I said. "What exactly do you do? Can I get a session with you?"

"Sounds are healing, dear," he said, referring to the beautiful chanting he had done the day before. "The ancient ones knew this. I could give you a Waitsu session down at the warm ponds if you'd like. There's a full moon coming up and that would be a perfect night to have a healing session, as the moon rises over the warm pond."

"What's Waitsu?" I asked.

"It's a form of Shiatsu, which is bodywork but done in water. I hold you as you float in the warm pond and then I gently pull and twist your body, your spine, your arms, and legs to move energy. Many people experience a release in emotions during the session as well. There are many health benefits to this type of work, especially in reducing chronic pain. I think it'd help you with the symptoms from the Lyme disease you were telling me about."

"Sounds perfect," I agreed.

Each day that I met up with Jacob, he would come up behind me and chant. Some days I would copy him and try to invite the healing in on a deeper level, and other days I would just relax and allow his sounds into my body. I imagined Dr. Emoto's work and pictured the beautiful images that were being created in my body as he sang.

Sitting under a tree one afternoon, he began chanting. It was mesmerizing. Curious about the language that he chanted in, I asked him.

"Now what language are you speaking? It sounds a bit different from the last time."

"It's Hebrew, love," he smiled.

On the night of the full moon, I met him at his house. We talked again about my experience with Lyme disease, and I told him something that I hadn't shared with anyone yet.

"I think I created this disease in my body." I awaited his response, but nothing came. "I had a near-death experience when I first arrived here on the island. I went to the light, and I met Jesus on the other side. I was shown the errors of my ways and mistakes that I have made with people. I saw how we create things in our life. I don't quite understand it all, but I'm learning."

He smiled and began to sing a familiar song. "*Mary did you know that your baby boy, would one day walk on water, Mary did you know…*" I leaned back and closed my eyes to listen. He had the most beautiful voice.

"Sing another," I pleaded when he finished the song.

He continued on and shifted into a chant while I took in the reverence of the sacred sounds. Darkness settled in and we got ready to go. We gathered some blankets and towels and headed out. As he drove, I texted Wendy to let her know

I would be late getting home. I also wanted her to know where I was, just in case. There was still a lingering fear that someone was following me.

There was one other car in the parking lot when we arrived. We made our way to the path that led to the water. The full moon was rising, illuminating the walkway. The evening air was comfortable even in my sundress. I had only known Jacob for two weeks and although we had connected, I was hesitant to completely trust him.

Following Jacob in the darkness, The Fear Miser began to crawl back into my mind with terrible images of being harmed. The voice tried to tell me that I was easy prey, that the darkness knew nothing, and it would not protect me.

I pushed the thoughts from my mind and began to hum. Trailing behind, Jacob led me to the side of the warm pond where I usually go. He stopped, set the backpack down, and pulled out the blankets to arrange them on the ground.

"I'm going to swim a bit, love," he sighed, looking up at the moon.

"Okay, I'll be in shortly," I said. "I want to sit here a bit and enjoy the stars." What I really needed was to feel comfortable again and get rid of the negative thoughts that kept trying to infiltrate. I laid back on the blanket and began to pray. I recited The Lord's Prayer in my mind and began to sing to myself. *"Jesus loves me this I know, for the Bible tells me so."* Suddenly like a little kid afraid of the dark, I chastised myself, got up, and walked to the water's edge.

I eased my way into the water. It felt warm and contrasted with the night air. Diving under, I swam down a bit to put my hands in the sandy bottom. When I came up for air, I turned to float on my back. The sky was brightly lit like a Christmas tree. Jacob swam up and supported my back with his arms. He told me to relax and close my eyes. When he began chanting, he took hold of one of my arms and began to move it in a circular motion while supporting me with his other arm. One way, and then another, he moved each arm until it became limp and allowed itself to be moved freely.

Next, he took hold of my wrists and began to swirl me around while he chanted. He moved down to my legs and did the same, moving them, stretching them, putting me into yoga-like positions, placing my body in a curled up fetal position, and then stretching me out to my fullest length.

He stopped chanting long enough to tell me to hold my breath, then he rolled me like a log, once, twice, then just as I was about to need air, he put his arms under me again and lifted my body out of the water. He instructed me to take a breath and hold it, so I floated effortlessly. Then letting go of me, he dove into the water to chant beneath me. Head to toe, I felt bubbles and the vibrations of his sounds while he moved underwater. In pure delight, almost ecstasy, peace and love filled me. I felt Oneness with the water, the sky, the air, and with Jacob. As he finished, he put his arms around me in a warm embrace and whispered words of Hebrew into my ear. "You are lovely, dear," he concluded, and then he let go and swam away.

~

When I finally arrived back at Wendy's, it was well after midnight. I climbed into bed too tired to write in my journal and slept like a baby until noon the next day. I awoke feeling like a new person.

I journaled my experience with Jacob then flipped back page by page reading several other entries about my near-death experience. I kept turning the pages, going backward in time, reading entries about Dr. P and entries from back in June and then May, and I noticed something. I was writing to God about a soul mate. At one point, I asked God to bring me a soul mate. Many entries began with "Dear God" or "Dear Universe" and then transitioned to "Dear Gail" instead.

At times, it was like I was writing to different beings, and other times it was like all beings were one and the same: me. Then I saw "Dear Soul Mate" and "My Dearest Love" as my greeting. The month before leaving for Maui, I was writing to my beloved and knew one day I would meet him.

As I sat and read through my journal, I remembered an author once instructed us to *act as if* something had already happened, and that would bring it into reality. Then, I remembered how some mornings I woke up thinking of a soul mate and began my day speaking to my beloved soul mate as if he were there waking up with me. I thought about waking up next to my beloved and kissing him good-bye when he left for work. I closed my eyes and began feeling all of my longings for health and happiness and love, but then I was interrupted by the sound of clinking glasses. Wendy walked into the bedroom with coffee.

"Hey, sweetie," she greeted me. "How was your night with Jacob?"

I shared with her about our talks and the healing session with him in the warm ponds. She listened for over an hour until my phone chirped.

I picked it up and saw a text message from Dr. P.

> I will be home in two weeks if you want to come back to Maui.

I replied.

> YES! I'd LOVE to come back!

He responded.

> I will call you when I return.

Grinning ear to ear, I bounced on the bed and told Wendy I was going to go back to Maui.

Later on, I called Jacob and told him I'd be leaving Big Island in a week or two and would have to focus on my writing until then. I thanked him for the Waitsu session and told him I needed to spend some time alone for the next day or two and would be in touch.

"What?" he objected. "Leaving already? Gee, love, I thought we'd have more time to spend together. Let me come get you. Just put away the writing and spend these last few days with me exploring some of the secret caverns that were on our list to do."

He was relentless until I gave in. "Give me a day or two," I said. "I'll see how I feel then. I just want time alone." I knew he was angry, but I didn't understand why. I promised I would call in two days, then hung up.

When the time came to call Jacob, I didn't want to. I wanted to keep writing. I wanted to dream about my month with T and I knew spending time with Jacob would only make matters more difficult when I left.

"Aloha, love," he greeted me. "I was just thinking about you."

"Aloha, Jacob" I replied. "I just put my computer away to take a walk outside and clear my head and thought I'd say hello."

"I'm going to one of the secret beaches that I told you about. Will you join me later? You'll love it there. There's big sea turtles swimming along the shoreline and small pools of water to soak in."

"I don't know, I'm not feeling it today," I said. I didn't want to go, but I didn't want to hurt his feelings.

"Oh, come on. It'll be our last hoorah and then I won't bug you anymore. Please, love."

"Where is this place? If it's not too far, I could meet you there." I didn't want to ride with him, and I had an uneasy feeling about going.

"I don't have a car today, I loaned mine to my roommate. What if you pick me up and I'll tell you where to go? It's not far. It's hard to explain how to get there because we have to park the car in a lot then hike along the coast."

I hesitated. My instincts said don't go. "Come on love," he persisted. "I gave you the Waitsu session; give me a few hours today."

I didn't want to go, but I caved. "Fine, Jacob. But just for a few hours. I need to be home before Wendy. We're going out for dinner tonight. I'll be down in half an hour. Be ready to go."

I couldn't tell you how we got to where we went, but I was instantly nervous when we stepped out of the car. Jacob told me to put all of my personal belongings in the trunk.

"If you leave anything visible, the windows are likely to get smashed and your belongings stolen," he cautioned.

It threw me off guard, that kind of negative warning, but I did as he said and put my stuff in the trunk. Grabbing my water bottle, I closed the trunk and the doors and locked the car behind me. It was nearing ninety-five degrees outside, and the sun was scorching hot.

Jacob had already begun his descent down the path when I realized I was still wearing flip-flops. He quickly turned and looked at me.

"We have to be back before five o'clock," he informed me. "After that, they lock the gate, and whatever cars are still inside here are stuck for the night."

"Well, I want to be back before Wendy," I reminded him nervously. "If it's an hour hike each way, let's just stop halfway whenever we see a good spot."

He made no sign of agreeing with me but instead began to sing and walk faster down the path of overgrown foliage and roots. I fell behind right away, tripping along the trail. We walked for maybe thirty minutes through fields and forests until we came across a creek. He finally stopped and let me catch up. Panting, I slugged some of my water down.

"I thought this was a hiking trail," I said to him. "I have no idea where we are. How are you going to find the way back to the car? We crisscrossed so many paths."

"No worry, love," he assured me. "I know the way. It's not much further. May I have a drink? I forgot my bottle in the car."

He nearly finished off the already half gone bottle of water then handed it back to me to take the last sip. I had become very unsettled and finally spoke up.

"Jacob, I don't feel so good. Can we just stop around here somewhere? Are we close to the ocean?"

He narrowed his eyes at me a bit, then motioned me to follow him. He cut through a thicket of branches and we traversed a gulley until finally the sky opened up to the sight of the ocean and my anxiety was relieved.

He made his way down the huge boulders and rock formations to where there were small pools of water filled with tiny tropical fish. He took off his clothes and entered one of the pools.

"Come join me!" he yelled.

"No thanks!" I said. "I want to see the turtles." Heading back up a large lava formation, I made my way to the top off a cliff. It was indeed a beautiful sight. There were half a dozen sea turtles coming into a cove. Delighted by the sight, I wanted to join them. I found my way down closer to the cove where I could get into a small pool of water in between the huge rocks.

Having left behind towels, bathing suits, and all my belongings in the car, I stripped down naked and stood atop the cliff. With my eyes softly closed and my arms stretched out to embrace the ocean, I tilted my head up to the sky. My heart expanded in complete surrender. I was a goddess, a timeless divine soul that had reached the point of reconnection in this lifetime.

When I entered the water, it felt heavenly, blissful. An hour must have passed before I heard Jacob. I looked up to see him climbing down the rocks.

"Is this a nude beach?" I called down to him, laughing. "Is nudity allowed anywhere on the island, or are we breaking rules?"

He slid in beside me and put his arm around me. "I just like being free," he said. Then leaning in, he planted a long kiss on my lips.

Pushing away, I stopped him. "Jacob, what are you doing?" I asked leaning back away from him.

I got up, got dressed, and headed back toward the tree line.

Jacob was behind me a few minutes later. "I'm sorry, love," he apologized. "Don't know what overcame me."

"Forget it," I laughed, trying to make light of it. "Just don't do it again."

Jacob wasn't laughing.

"Which way do we go to get out of here?" I asked. "It must be getting close to the time that we need to head back. I don't want Wendy's car locked inside the gates."

He took off without another word. Back through the thickets, across a stream and gulley before he stopped to look at me.

"Give me the keys and I'll run ahead," he said in a rush. "I'll sit with the car in case the county guys come to lock up the gate."

My intuition told me not to give him the keys, but I did it anyway. He grabbed them and ran. I immediately scolded myself. Not only did he have the keys to the car, but he had access to my purse with my credit cards, passport, and driver's license. I suddenly became afraid I'd lose my way back. My mind started wandering, wondering if he had planned this all along. *Was he sending someone back here to hurt me?* I wondered. No one knew where I was.

My mind ran wild. I began reciting The Lord's Prayer as I was completely overridden with fear. I started to run but tripped over tree roots and rocks, stumbled, and fell. There were two men walking down the path towards me. In a panic, I tried to call Wendy on my phone but had no service, so I spoke into the phone as if having a conversation with someone.

"No, Mom," I said loud enough for the men to hear. "I'm heading back to the car. I have to be to work in an hour, but I'll try to stop by on my way. Anything else you need at the drug store?"

I paused as if she would answer.

"Yes, yes, I know. Jacob ran out of water, so I shared mine with him."

As the two men approached, I smiled and kept talking as if someone was really on the phone. I exchanged a friendly "Aloha" with the men as they passed by, then I resumed my fake conversation about turtles and the weather. I picked up my pace and didn't look back until I knew they were out of sight. I ran the rest of the way until, panting, I saw Jacob sitting in the car with the air conditioning on.

"Did you see the guys that headed out on the path?" I asked.

"What guys?" he asked. "No, I didn't see anyone."

~

That was the last day I saw or called Jacob. I spent the following days writing and walking around Wendy's yard contemplating our fearsome trek, wondering if he was going to hurt me or if my own fears had put those strange men on my path. If our thoughts truly created our reality, then I created those men. I felt like I was in the twilight zone, wondering if they had even been real.

Over the next two weeks, I spent less time exploring the island and more time writing and reflecting. I focused on my book and daily health routines. In the mornings, I wrote on the lanai. At night, I journaled letters to my soul mate. I spent much of my thoughts on my health and P and kept researching the healing benefits of the waters of Hawaii and augmenting my own theories.

Wendy had reserved a spot for us in a class with a Hawaiian shaman. He was teaching about heart-centered shamanism at a place just down on Kalapana Road. We planned our last couple of days together to include the class and an afternoon at an ecstatic dance class. I was making the most of every day, but I was eagerly counting down the days until P got home.

We were cooking dinner one night when my phone rang. It was P.

"Good morning, P!" I shouted excitedly. I loved the way P said good morning no matter what time of day it was.

"Good morning," he chuckled. "How are you?"

"I'm great! I'm so happy to hear from you! Are you back in Maui? How are you feeling?"

"Yes, I'm back, feeling a bit tired from the long flights, but other than that, I'm doing okay. Do you still want to come over?"

"Yes!" I about hollered.

"Okay," he laughed. "When is good for you?"

My eyes widened as he opened the door for any possibility. "I'm ready to come over now," I joked.

"Okay, well, why don't you look at flights for the next day or two and let me know when you can come."

Wide-eyed, I looked at Wendy and repeated it loudly for her to hear. "Really? I can come *now*? I plan to stay until I have to leave and go back to New York at the end of August. How long do you want me there? If I come in the next day or two, that means I'll be there for almost a month," I laughed. "Are you sure you want me there for that long?" I was praying he would say yes. Wendy's eyes grew as did mine.

"Well, I haven't thought about it," P said. "But why not? You may hate me by the end of that time, but you can come stay as long as you want."

"Wonderful! I'll look at flights tonight and let you know what day I can fly over."

The thought of seeing P again consumed me. I was going back to Maui! What would my family say to me, staying with this stranger, with this Iranian doctor that I just met in Buffalo? *People will think I'm crazy*, I thought. I wanted to follow my heart, to follow the bliss, but there was a conditioned part of me that was afraid.

I could feel these two energies in me, light and dark. They were having a field day with me. The one was full of adventure, full of life and new beginnings. This was the light and love that I felt towards this man. This was the part of me that screamed yes and told me to go. The other heavy, dark side that lurked in the background weighed on my fears and doubts and past hurts and abandonment. This was the part that nudged negative thoughts into my consciousness and asked me if I dared, the part that questioned my sanity, the part that told me it was not safe to trust.

I sent a text message to Mary.

> P said I can come anytime. I'm afraid. I don't know why. I hate being afraid.

She texted back.

> Jeremiah 29:11

I opened the internet on my phone and searched the verse: "For I know the plans I have for you, declares the Lord, plans to prosper you and not harm you, plans to give you hope and a future."

I messaged Mary back.

> Thank you!

That settled it. I knew I had to go. I pulled out my computer and searched flights to Maui. There were only two flights to choose from. I read the flight details aloud to Wendy and asked her which one to book.

"Really, Gail," she rolled her eyes with a smile. "Flight 111! What does *that* tell you? In numerology, the Universe speaks in angel numbers to tell you when to pay attention. That's how you stay focused on the positive because a lot of good things are coming your way!"

With that, I booked the flight. Giddy as a schoolgirl, I called P back and told him I'd be there that Sunday then hung up the phone and danced around the kitchen.

I turned and looked at Wendy smiling ear to ear. "Gail Lynn, you better go shopping tomorrow and get a new dress!" she said. "You want to greet that Dr. P in something cute. You're going to be good for him just like he has been good for you! Maybe *he* is the love you've been looking for."

I giggled as I thought about my journal. Of course, I wondered the exact same thing.

~

Lao Tzu once said, "Being deeply loved by someone gives you strength while loving someone deeply gives you courage."

~

The next day I spent hours shopping for dresses, earrings, shoes, a purse, a bathing suit, and a nightgown. I was pleased with my purchases. Living with a man for the next month was going to be different. I poured a glass of wine for Wendy and me that night at dinner and showed her my new wardrobe.

"You're glowing," she noted. "You're happy and healthy. I'm glad you are finally taking care of *you*."

I fell asleep happy that night, wondering where life was going to lead me this next month. I felt like I was playing out my own version of the board game Life, rolling the dice and taking chances.

~

Saturday was my last day with Wendy. We spent the day together walking around the yard, having heart to heart talks about everything from my early childhood traumas and relationship and trust issues to sickness and the stress brought on by my employer. We talked about the near-death experience and all of the healing opportunities I had. The warm ponds, the singing bowls, the chanting with Jacob, and the class with the Shaman had all helped me along my journey. Going back to Maui seemed like the natural next step in the divine plan of my life, and I couldn't wait to arrive at my next destination. I tried to capture it on the page that night as I wrote in my journal.

July 29th, 2017
Dearest Beloved,
Today was my last day on the Big Island. It marks an end, but also a beginning. I have many fears, but I ask God, Source, to shed some light on the pathway that begins tomorrow. Oh God, take away the fears and bring wisdom and courage. Instead, lead me to the right path for my highest and best. Take away negative energies and people who wish to do me harm. Surround me with all the angels. I am grateful for this day and the next part of my adventure. My dear soulmate, my heart flutters with excitement to meet you again. We have a great story to tell of East meets West. Sleep well, my love.
G~

~

Wendy drove me to the airport the next morning, and we said goodbye. I went to the gate to wait. I was staring out the window at the tarmac when my phone rang.

"Hi, Momma!" I answered.

"Hi, sweetie! How's it going? Where are you?"

"Well," I drawled it out, we had a lot to catch up on. "I'm at the airport on Big Island. I'm heading over to Maui for the remainder of my summer. I'm going to stay with Dr. P, the man I met while boarding the airplane in Buffalo."

"What?" she was shocked. "Sweetie, are you sure you know what you're doing? You hardly know the man. How do you know he's not a murderer?" Her voice dripped with concern.

"Mom! Stop! You watch too much TV," I didn't want to get into it with her. "I don't know why I need to go, but I do. Stop being a worrywart. And stop being so negative. Will you please just see it in your mind that everything goes smoothly. You have to picture amazing things happening.

What if your negative thoughts put me in harm's way? Dr. P is a kind, loving person. I'll call you when I land in Maui."

I hung up before I could give her another opportunity to plant a negative thought in my mind. I got in line to board Flight 111 to Maui. I recapped all the ways the angels got our attention. I settled into my seat, put my headphones on, and pulled up a podcast. A quick internet search of the spiritual meaning of the number 111 told me that this number was a sign from the angels that our thoughts are manifesting instantly. I wasn't surprised. Denise and I had manifested those last two nights with P, thinking about how lovely it would be to spend time with him. I closed my eyes and pictured good things happening.

The plane landed right on time. A little more than four weeks had passed since I had seen P. I turned on my phone and heard the chirp of a text.

It was from P.

Welcome to Maui.

My heart fluttered.

Home sweet home.

~13~

Love, The Healing Elixir

Before getting my luggage, I stopped at the washroom to freshen up. I felt the butterflies begin to swirl. The giddiness escaped as I smoothed out my dress. I stood at the basin washing my hands and turned to the woman beside me.

"It's a good day," I said cheerfully.

I grabbed my luggage and headed out to the curb. P called to say he was coming around the parking loop and would be there in a few minutes. Closing my eyes and turning my head to the sun-streaked sky, I took a deep breath and allowed my thoughts to flow in and out. It was still difficult to believe that I was in Maui and on my way to stay with an Iranian doctor who had opened up his heart and home to me. My thoughts drifted to the television news and war with Iran and I wondered, *Why don't the news stations tell Americans how beautiful and compassionate the Iranian people are?* Then I remembered T's wave of the hand when I asked how to pronounce his name and inquired what his lineage was. What if the world COULD see his people differently? What if he and I, the Middle East and the

American West, were here to show the world a different story? My heart smiled at that thought.

Hearing a car pull up, I opened my eyes. I made out the silhouette through the car window. I noticed his hair was a little shorter now with hints of burgundy. His smile made my heart skip a beat as he got out of the car, walked over to me, and wrapped his arms around me in a warm embrace.

"Good morning, how was your flight?" I smiled at P's familiar greeting. *We've done this before*, I thought. I breathed in his scent and savored the moment. The smell of his cologne tickled my nose. I hugged him tighter, thrilled to be back in Maui with him.

"It's so good to see you!" I blushed.

"Get in the car where it's cooler," he said, grabbing my bags.

I slid into the front seat and welcomed the blast of cool air, a relief from the Maui heat. It was already peaking at ninety degrees, and it wasn't even noon. P got in and looked at me as he shifted into drive.

"You look good," he smiled. It felt nice to be given a compliment from this man I admired. I had butterflies in my stomach. My mind raced with so many thoughts. I wanted to get my words right. I was a small-town girl trying to find her way in a world of travelers.

"Thank you, P. You look good, too. I'm so excited to be here again. Thank you for the invitation to come back." I watched him stare straight ahead, smiling, nodding. I still found it hard to believe that I was there, back in Maui, sitting next to P again.

"I have to go into work for a few hours," P said. "You can take the car and explore a little until I'm done. Have you eaten? There are a few nice restaurants in the area and there is an organic store close by as well if you need to grab a bite."

"Yes, I'm starving," I replied. "I'll find a little coffee shop or something and then head to a beach somewhere to sit and write."

"There are many fine beaches here in Kihei. Just drive down the road and you'll see one after another."

"Perfect. I can't wait to get in the water. After you're done with work, will you swim with me?"

P chuckled. "No thank you. It's been a while since I've been in the ocean. You go ahead. How was Big Island?"

My thoughts shifted to the past four weeks. My smile slipped away at the memory of being at death's front door. I didn't want to tell him about the pass from Jacob or the fear that I had about someone harming me. It all seemed like lifetimes ago, and I just wanted to create good things while here with him on Maui.

"Big Island was good," I answered. "We went to the warm ponds, went snorkeling, picked up a few hitchhikers, and then Wendy's nieces came to visit." I laughed at the memory of picking up a hitchhiker. I had changed so much.

"We went to Waikiki and Pearl Harbor. There's so much history there. I cried as I walked the grounds. And when we boarded a submarine for a tour, I was overcome with so much emotion that I couldn't continue; I had to get off the submarine. A strange feeling came over me as if I had been there before. I went and sat on a bench and closed my eyes. Visons passed through my mind of open fields and a girl running. She fell when a bomb exploded a short distance away from her. Then a man came and picked her up and held her in his arms. She died. It was all very odd." Contemplating my next question, I asked hesitantly, "Do you believe in past lives?"

He turned and looked out the window to the ocean as we drove the coastline. "No," he said.

I skipped over telling him about the near-death experience on the night I almost died. Then I thought to myself, *Perhaps I did die, and this is all a dream.*

Wanting to change the subject, I looked at P to gauge his health. Last month he said he was recovering from a procedure, and I wanted to ask about his health without digging too much.

"What about you? How is your healing going?"

He just smiled and nodded. "I'm good." We arrived at his office and I hopped into the driver's seat. "You could come in and sit in my office while I see patients," he said, "but you'd probably have more fun at the beach. I'll give you a call when I'm done for the day." He took a long look into my eyes. "I'm glad you're here," he said leaning down and gently brushing my cheek with a kiss.

The nervousness dissipated as I planted a kiss on his cheek in return. "I'm glad I'm here, too," I said. Smiling ear to ear, P turned and walked towards the door with easy strides. I looked up at the clear, blue sky feeling bliss.

Dear God, thank you.

I got back in the car, buckled myself in, and spoke aloud to my angels. "Spirit lead me!" I declared.

As I drove, observing the blue and green shades of the ocean, I felt happier than ever. I rolled down the windows and breathed in the fresh ocean air. I turned up the radio as I drove no more than a mile before coming to a large parking lot. I pulled in, put the car in park, grabbed my backpack that held my laptop and journal, and ran like a child to the beach. I dropped my bag in the sand, kicked off my sandals, and went straight to the water.

I snapped a photo of my toes in the water to text to P.

I'm in!

He responded with a smile.

For the next hour, I walked in ecstasy along the shore, stopping to stare out into the dazzling blue waters. I felt great peace. I was home. *P* was home.

When I had my fill of walking, I went back to my towel and pulled out my journal. Feeling nostalgic, I began flipping through the pages to read the thoughts I had recorded. As if my angels guided me where to start, I opened to the days right before leaving New York.

June 17, 2017

Good morning my love, only a few more days! I can't wait to be in your arms, hold you, touch you, kiss you, love you ~ I am...

My reminiscing was interrupted by a phone call from P to let me know he was free to leave for the day. I was ecstatic.

He was waiting outside for me when I pulled in, his quiet charm, the gentle smile, pulling at my heart. I got out to give him a quick kiss on the cheek before getting back into the passenger seat. It was so good to be here; I couldn't stop telling him.

The car ride along the coast up to Lahaina was breathtaking. I was in awe at the way the sun danced on the waves of the Pacific as if millions of diamonds were moving to the song of the sea. The blue-green water and the palm trees swaying in the afternoon breeze filled my heart.

I struggled with finding the right words to say, so I said what came to my mind. "There is something about being here on the island of Maui with you that fills my heart with such joy! Thank you," I tried. "Really, thank you."

He turned and looked at me with gentle eyes. "You're welcome." A man of few words, always deep in thought, P stared ahead as he drove.

A few minutes later we passed by a beach with snorkelers, and I told him I wanted to try. "Will you go with me sometime?" I asked. "Are you ready to get into the ocean with me?"

My body was craving a dive into the ocean to absorb all the yummy minerals. He didn't answer, but instead laughed and accelerated around the curves and cliffs that stretched along the highway. Although his demeanor was steadfast and calm, he had an adventurous spirit that always liked to push the limits of life. Just another trait I found admirable, living life to the fullest. Recalling the ride in his Corvette last month, hitting speeds over 100 mph between lights, I wasn't sure if he was trying to impress me with his bravery or testing my courage.

As we turned off the highway to head up the mountain, I could see the entrance gate to his property. We were welcomed once again by Buddha. I smiled, home sweet home.

He brought my luggage inside to my bedroom, the same room Denise and I shared the previous month. The beautiful room with the king-sized bed and lounge chair had the best view of the ocean. The wall of massive sliding glass doors allowed the sun to enter each morning and the dazzling sunsets each night.

After I settled in and hung up my clothes, I walked back outside to the lanai where the infinity pool and hot tub were. I smiled taking it all in. Then I remembered his health and wondered how his healing was going, considering all of his travels.

Hearing his footsteps behind me, I looked back and saw him holding a towel. "Why don't you go for a swim? I wasn't sure if there were extra towels in your room, but here's one for you."

"Will you come in with me?" I begged. He just laughed and walked over to place his hand in the water and feel its temperature.

"I'll keep you company from the patio sofa. It's quite comfortable, and the kitties need my attention. They hate it when I am gone for so long." Just then, Cleo and Boy walked over to him and began rubbing up against his leg.

"CLEO! BOY!" I exclaimed excitedly. "It's so good to see you again." I went over and gave them each a kiss on the top of their heads then turned to P. "Okay, but what about the hot tub? You up for that?"

"Now *that* I can do. I'll get it heating. Are you hungry? I don't have much here, but we can go to Costco in the morning for groceries." He walked over to the switch box on the wall and turned on the jacuzzi. "How about a glass of wine?"

I began to lift the sundress up over my head. "Sounds perfect." I dove into the pool and swam the length in one breath. I was more than satisfied. *Progress*, I thought.

The sun began setting and another elegant display of beauty began. I swam a few more laps then noticed P watching me. I got out of the pool, grabbed a towel, and joined him on the sofa. He handed me a glass of wine, and clinking glasses, we toasted to another beautiful sunset.

We sat and watched the sky until the sun disappeared below the horizon.

"Tell me," he said, "did you have any symptoms arise while you were on Big Island?"

"I've been feeling really good actually. I've been eating healthy foods. I spent time in the warm ponds and have been learning about the health benefits of minerals like sulfur in the water. I think my body was missing these minerals. I'm still using essential oils, too. Wendy kept me occupied, sending me on explorations."

I paused to consider the significance of that.

"I didn't have time to think about being sick," I said.

Then my mind went to the night I died in Wendy's arms and the thought that my Living Will was sitting on my kitchen counter. A shiver ran up my spine. The vision of Jesus standing over me, reaching out with his two fingers, touching me was etched in my mind. I didn't want to tell P about any of that. He probably wouldn't have believed me.

Trying to divert the conversation, I walked back to the pool and dove into the crystal blue water. That was how I avoided having to participate in a difficult conversation.

His voice interrupted my thoughts. "The hot tub should be warm by now."

"Are *you* ready?" I asked

He walked over to the chaise and with one hand on the back of the chair, he slid his blue hospital scrubs down. Using his feet, he pushed one pant leg off and then the other. Standing there fully naked, my eyes stared in surprise before blushing and turning away. Looking up at the starry sky, my mind began reeling with thoughts and questions. I was not used to his ways and I was at a loss for words again.

P stepped into the steamy water and paused on the first step just as I was pulling myself up out of the pool to ease myself into the hot tub. It gave me a direct line of vision to the scar that remained from his procedure. He took another step and then sunk down until his whole body was submerged. I wondered if it was the heat or the scar that caused the grimace on his face, but I pretended not to notice. Instead, I pointed to the North Star. Just as I opened my mouth to name it, a shooting star streaked the sky.

"Look!" I squealed with joy. "Make a wish!"

His eyes scanned the twinkling diamonds above. I wondered what he was wishing for. I wished for his health to improve.

Leaning back, he closed his eyes and smiled, stretched his legs out across the seat, and rested them against mine. I reached down with my hand and grabbed one of his feet. That same spark of familiarity shot through me. *We've done this before*, came the voice in my head.

He pointed out some of the star systems before sitting back and getting lost in thought. My mind wandered to the day we were taken off the plane in Buffalo and the sudden closeness that I felt toward him. I thought about the meditation I did in Wendy's yard on Big Island under the moon. The vision appeared again of a dusty road below a crumbled building and feet sticking out from underneath the pile of rubble. I shook the thought from my mind and returned to the present moment. Looking at him from my peripheral vision, I tried speaking to him telepathically.

Why are you so familiar to me?

As if not wanting to answer, he said, "My body has had enough heat. I'll pour us some wine."

I responded to his change of conversation. "Okay, that sounds good!" He either ignored my thought on purpose or wasn't aware of the thoughts I sent him. I stared after him admiring his confidence and his nakedness and sent him another question in my thoughts. *Are you in pain, P?* But again, no reply. When he returned with the wine glasses, he set them down on the table and then adjusted the towel around his waist.

"You sure look good without any clothes on," I joked, still not quite used to all the nakedness.

As always, uncomfortable with a compliment, he commented on his age and weight, putting himself down.

I hated that he did that. "You shouldn't be so hard on yourself, P. You're a handsome man." I tried again to let him know I really admired his sun-kissed body as much as his wit and intelligence. My words always failed. Looking up at the evening sky, I closed my eyes and took a deep breath.

"What did I do to deserve all this grandeur?" I whispered aloud. No response came. My throat tightened as emotions rose. I couldn't identify the feeling. Is this love? Compassion? Familiarity? Was it a past life reawakened? All of it flowed through my mind as if on a movie reel. Wayne Dyer, Polynesian Islands, Mediterranean Sea, Galilee…

"Are you thirsty?" P's voice broke through the movie in my mind. I climbed out of the hot tub, wrapped up in the towel he had laid out for me, and reached for the glass of wine he held out.

"Cheers," he said.

"To a month of writing, healing, laughter, and adventure!" I said.

"Yes, to all that," he laughed.

I walked out from under the cover of the lanai to where I could see the stars. My hand went to my heart to feel it beating wildly. I told myself it was all okay, that it would all be okay. Every time I looked at him, my heart felt like it was growing bigger, cracking, opening.

I know you. Who are you?

My soul knew his soul.

"Would you like to watch a movie?" he asked. "Have you seen *The Notebook*? It's a beautiful story."

"Yes!" I answered laughing. "And yes, I would like to watch it. It's been a long time since I've seen it. I don't remember much about it. Is it a story about a writer?" I laughed. I could remember scenes but not titles.

"We should watch it," he smiled and refilled our glasses.

We sat down on the sofa and settled in. We clinked glasses once more as if to initiate our month of August together. I was happier than I had been in a long time. There was absolutely no thought of illness, symptoms, fear, bullying, hospitals, inflammation, or pain. We watched and giggled at the young lovers on the big screen TV. Then P set his glass down and placed his hand on my leg. Like long lost lovers, we nestled up together. It felt right, natural as if I had done it before.

Watching the characters play out their roles, love filled the air. P reached for his wine, finished it in a gulp, then stretched his legs around behind me, pulling me down to lay beside him. I savored the moment with his arm wrapped around me again. It had been a long time since I felt close to someone, felt this feeling of being unconditionally accepted, protected, cared for. Perhaps P needed this, too.

I don't know how much time passed, but the sound of shouting voices on the TV startled me awake. I had fallen asleep. His light snoring told me he was fast asleep as well. Feeling my legs weighted down by his legs intertwined with mine, I smiled. What a good feeling it was to be held.

I didn't want to stir or wake him, but my arm had tingles running up to my shoulder. I wanted to stay like that all night, but my movement woke him.

"Good morning," he whispered.

"So much for watching the movie," I giggled.

"I'll rewind it. It's a good movie. You should see it." He sat up and lit a cigarette then grabbed the remote. "Shall I get another?" he asked, pointing at the empty wine bottle with a grin.

I grabbed the empty bottle and headed for the kitchen. "Pinot Noir or Merlot?" I asked.

There was no answer, so I opened the Pinot Noir and went back to the sofa. I welcomed the loss of fear and inhibition that came with each glass of wine. I could get out of my head and be myself without self-judgment or self-condemnation.

Setting the glasses down on the coffee table, I glanced out at the pool. "First a midnight swim?" I tried.

"You go ahead. I'll finish my cigarette. I have to make a quick call to my family in Iran. We can restart the movie after that."

He stood and walked to the other room and I walked out to the pool. Relaxed and free, I dropped the towel still wrapped around me. Accepting myself in all my flaws, I stretched out my arms, my body naked and free of self-doubt, I reached for the stars.

"I love you, Maui!" I shouted.

I dove in eager to make the lap, pushing myself to go even further this time. When I finally came up for air, I felt energized. I swam over to the edge where the water spilled off into infinity and looked out to the grand pacific. It was heaven here. I sighed and rested my head on my arms, closed my eyes, and allowed a dream to come. My imagination ran wild as I pictured what it would be like to wake up here every day.

"Counting stars?" he asked, interrupting my thoughts. I turned and swam to him.

"Not counting," I said, "but wishing upon them."

I started to climb the stairs to get out, but the night breeze reminded me of my nakedness and a shiver prompted P to hand me a towel.

"It's 78 degrees," he laughed. "How can you be cold?" He wrapped me in another towel then handed me the glass of wine. "This should help you warm up, too."

We went back inside to restart the movie.

After a sip, I set my glass down on the table and leaned back into P again.

"Here," he said, laying a pillow on his arm. "This will be more comfortable than my arm." He gently pulled me in to lay back down beside him. Wrapped in towels, I laced my legs between his. Between laughter and tears, we finished the movie and fell asleep in each other's arms. We stayed like that on the sofa until the roosters crowed and the sun began to rise.

I awoke thinking about my dream, of being kissed passionately and losing all inhibition with P. Then I noticed that the towel that was wrapped around me, was now on the floor. Boy was laying on the back of the sofa softly purring, occasionally blinking at me. Cleo was sitting upright on the coffee table staring as if telling me it was time to get up. Whether a dream or a dreaming reality, somewhere in my sleep we had caressed each other for the simple enjoyment that came from unconditional love, healing love.

Watching the clock on the DVD player, I lay quietly in the pleasure of being held. It was 6:00 am when my body began prompting me to move. I carefully lifted P's arms and snuck away to shower, dress, and sit on the lanai to write. Two hours passed before I realized P was supposed to go to work. I went inside and stood over him, quietly calling out his name, but he didn't move. I began caressing his head and rubbing the day-old whiskers on his cheek.

His eyes fluttered open. Looking up at me still dreamy, he suddenly sat up. "What time is it?" he asked. Reaching for his phone and heading into his bedroom, I heard him call his secretary. "I'll be there in 20 minutes."

I made his coffee and set his keys out for him to find.

Minutes later he walked into the kitchen. "You look handsome. And you smell good, too. Do you need anything for lunch?"

He sipped his coffee and picked up his keys. "I don't eat lunch," he said smiling. "But thank you." He handed me a second set of car keys. "Go have fun today. Explore the island. I should be home around five o'clock." He planted a kiss on my cheek then headed out the door.

I had no desire to leave the house. My heart was full. I sat on the lanai, played with Cleo and Boy, and worked on my manuscript. I took breaks to walk up the back mountain to the Buddha garden and meditate. Writing, swimming, meditating; my afternoon was full of things that made my heart smile. I wanted to share all this with someone.

I called Mary and told her about my first day back with P. "My heart feels so happy here like I'm home," I told her. "Mary, love is the healing medicine I needed." I recapped my first night back with P.

"*The Notebook*?" she asked laughing.

"What?" I asked. "What's wrong with *The Notebook*?"

"You've been *Notebook*ed and don't even know it!"

"I don't know what that means, but I *do* know that it was a really good night."

I cleaned the house, cut some fresh flowers for the table, and told Alexa to play some jazz music. The house was coming alive again. As if she had feelings of her own, I went about the house all day adjusting things, shifting the energy to liven things up. In the kitchen, I was wiping down the windowsill when I came across a plaque. It read:

Never
Never
Never
Give up

Interesting, I thought. Someone at some time thought this was important advice to give to P, or, he bought it as a reminder to himself. Perhaps it was true, what I was feeling, that we needed each other. *Is this what is meant by "like attracts like"*? I wondered.

When P got home, we decided to go for groceries.

"If we go to Costco, we can get a slice of pizza and share a Pepsi before shopping. The roosters there are fun to watch." The simple pleasure of conversation, laughter, and being in paradise was enough.

When we arrived back home, he suggested another movie. *Avatar*. After putting groceries away, I jumped in the pool to swim a few laps while he popped the cork on a bottle of Merlot. I could tell he was still avoiding the water, so I didn't bring up the hot tub. The movie led to greater conversations, pausing at times to discuss the relevancy. We fell asleep again with our legs interlocked, his arms pulling me close.

Each morning before heading off to work, P suggested I play and explore Maui just like Wendy had done. The first couple of days, I stuck by the house, writing, swimming in the pool, and being entertained by the silly antics of Boy and Cleo. After a few days, I began to venture outside of his home. First, it was to the beach park within minutes of his home. After a few more days passed, I began driving further north, exploring Ka'anapali, the area where my favorite author Wayne Dyer used to live.

Going off on my own one morning, as I drove the winding roads of the upper part of the island, a feeling of melancholy overcame me. That inner voice began talking to me again and said, *I don't want to explore alone anymore. I want to share these adventures with someone. I want to share my life with someone.*

Later that night, when P got home, I told him that. He just nodded his head in quiet contemplation, avoiding eye contact. Nothing more was said, but I picked up on what *wasn't* said. I turned in for bed early that night, closed my bedroom door behind me, and sat on my bed to write.

~

Two weeks had passed, and the adventures, although beautiful and appreciated, were not as meaningful anymore. I was lonely exploring on my own. We still watched movies together, but I began sleeping in my own bedroom at night. Watching others explore the island with their companions struck a nerve with me. Here I was on the beautiful, romantic island of Maui, and I felt lonely. I had no one to share it with.

It was shortly after midnight one night when I heard P's voice coming from the other room. He was yelling. I got up and went to the bedroom door to open it and see what he wanted, but soon realized he was talking on the phone and not calling out to me. He was speaking another language.

The next morning, I heard the TV blaring, so I went out to see what was going on. He stood watching the news as headlines scrolled across the bottom of the TV. North Korea was threatening military attacks. I turned away, avoiding the bad news. *Ho'oponopono*, I thought.

"Why do you watch this negative stuff, P?"

"It's important to know what's going on in the world. You should pay attention," he responded.

"No thanks. I have not had a TV in my house for almost two years. If I want to see a movie, I'll play a DVD. Everything on TV is negative news. They program people to always see the bad in everything." I turned to walk away, but his next words stopped me in my tracks.

"Well, it's affecting my business. I have to go away for ten days. I am having some work done on a house over in Iran and need to make some decisions. I'll be leaving Friday. Cleo and Boy will keep you company while I'm away."

My heart practically stopped.

"What do you mean you have to go away? Seriously?" My mind raced with questions and The Fear Miser returned in full force. He explained again trying to make it sound as if being away for ten days was nothing, but he did not understand me. He did not understand my fears. *How could he leave me*? My inner child screamed.

Later that evening after our fill of *Star Trek* episodes, I said good night and went to my bedroom to write.

Contemplating the day's events, I wondered how the news of Korea could affect his business. I pulled up Korea on a map and meditated on the country, sending love and healing to the people. I snapped a picture of it and wrote the words "Ho'oponopono" across the map. Then I pulled out my journal and began writing.

Dear Korea,
I'm sorry. Please forgive me. Thank you. I love you.

~

The next two days flashed by quickly. There was so much that I wanted to say to him before he left, but my fear of rejection and abandonment were at the forefront of my mind. I didn't feel safe sharing my feelings with him. As usual, the voice inside reminded me it would only open me up to rejection. This voice beckoned me into a paralyzed silence that was reminiscent of my childhood.

When the day arrived to take him to the airport, I felt ill. I didn't tell him though. I didn't want to appear weak. We barely spoke on the ride to the airport. I didn't know what to say, so I stared out the window instead. The trapped energy and emotion tried to escape in tears, but I forced those to stay inside, too. My throat tightened, my chest felt heavy. We pulled up, got out, and he turned to me to brush his lips gently across my cheek in a kiss goodbye.

"I'll see you in ten days," he said.

"Okay," I whispered. "Be safe." I could barely speak. I was left standing at the curb wondering what was happening, feeling afraid and abandoned again.

The little girl inside began to scream at me.

I told you so. I told you he would leave you, too.

~14~

Face Your Fears

Driving back to the house in confusion, I reprimanded myself for caring about P so much. War raged inside me. All of the fear of abandonment came to the forefront of my mind. I should've known better than to get my emotions wrapped up in this person, in this *thing* I had going on with this man. Last month he was just a stranger on a plane. I came to Maui to heal, to find solutions, and write my book about healing holistically. What I found though was something even greater. I found a stirring in my heart again that resembled something called love.

He saved my job, showed me compassion, and opened my heart to love again, but where was he now? I didn't think I'd ever love again, but he changed that. Something within me had changed. I wanted love again. How dare he! How dare he be so kind and loving only to leave me.

The house was dark and quiet, fitting. I stood in the open doorway and gazed around the room, that great room with all the windows looking out to the Pacific. It was so quiet, eerie. My home, a place of respite, yet suddenly I felt afraid. My mind began playing tricks on me. I felt an enemy hiding around the corner waiting to ambush me, and I dreaded the next ten days.

A vision first came to me in a dream. A nightmare, rather. I knew I shouldn't focus on it, as I didn't want to bring it into my reality. I intentionally turned my thoughts to other things. I spent several days at the beach, driving around the island and exploring. I spent a whole day cleaning the house. I scrubbed the floors as I fought to forget about P, but my thoughts kept returning back to him.

Someone once told me an old proverb, "What you resist, persists." I contemplated that thought and many others from great mystical teachers that appeared in my stream of consciousness.

One morning while sitting in meditation, I saw a large beige stone, and beyond that an entrance to a cave. I heard the words, *Make a decision.* A deep chill ran through my bones. I forced it out of my head. Then I saw P wrapped up in ropes, tied to a chair with his head dropped down to his chest. I didn't know where these images came from, but they played out in my mind during my meditation until I finally quit.

Empty your mind, Gail, I told myself. *It's not real. Focus on what you want, not on false images. False Evidence Appearing Real is how the mind tricks us.*

I called Mary for help. "Please tell me these visions I'm having of P are not real," I begged. "I've been meditating, Mary, or trying to, but scary visions keep popping into my head."

"What's going on?" she asked. "Of course you can change your visions, Gail, but free will keeps you from interfering in other people's choices."

"The law of attraction says that I can manifest how I want things to go. Can't I just envision P being safe and returning? I'm seeing awful visions in my head of him getting hurt! It's scaring me and I'm here alone."

"Stay in the vortex, Gail. Change your thoughts and create the reality that you want. You will know by August 20 what is happening."

"What? What do you mean? Why the 20th?"

"I don't know. You are the one with the gift. I just keep seeing that day as significant. You will know something by then, and for the sake of being prepared, you may want to find another way to the airport when you leave."

"WHAT? What does that mean? Mary, you think he's not coming back?? WHY?"

I didn't know what to think but then Mary said she had to go.

We hung up and I began pacing the floor until Cleo and Boy started to circle around me. The rest of the afternoon was spent writing, swimming in the pool, and watering the gardens. I started getting hungry, so I headed to the kitchen to find something to create for dinner, but two large centipedes were racing to beat me there.

Even the critters are closing in on me, I thought. That's all I need is to step on one of them and end up in the hospital without P here to take care of me. I decided to start a movie and fall asleep on the sofa.

The next day, I woke up early and went to Kihei to see my friend, Kate. I wasn't sure if I wanted to share with her my fears or not. We decided to drive the famous Road to Hana, so we quickly packed some snacks and water bottles and headed out.

Kate brought along her *Maui Revealed* guidebook and highlighted all the waterfalls we would stop to see. At each mile marker, I was eager to see what marvelous sight was waiting in the thick of bamboo and forests. At each area, we swam in the waterfalls and hiked through the mud. A recent rain brought enough water to overflow the creeks and flood many of the paths.

Each waterfall was more beautiful than the last. The water was healing. The air was clean, crisp, and light. At one point, I sat under the falls allowing the water to pour over my head and asking Goddess Pele and the Spirits of Hawaii to cleanse me of any fear or negativity. I pictured my energy being cleansed like I was whole again, and peace washed over me.

"Thank you, Maui, for sharing your beauty with me," I said beneath the waterfall. I felt the love of Maui wrap around me.

Continuing communication with the spirit world, I prayed for answers. I prayed to know why I was endlessly tested. I prayed to know the connection between fear and loneliness. I prayed to know what love was and what the connection was between P and me. I looked to the clouds, awaiting a reply. The sun warmed my face. I waited. Nothing came. I left the water and sat down with Kate, together we stared at the sky and chatted mindlessly about everything and nothing.

Our next spot to explore brought us to meet two little girls, ages eight and ten. They were heading down a natural path of lava smoothed over by the crashing waves of water. I watched them as the older one jumped in. The younger of the two stood waiting for the ocean waves to calm down. That is when Spirit spoke to me.

Tell her to speak to the water.

I stood watching her and then heard the voice in my head again.

Tell her to speak to the water. Respect the water and the water will respect you. Tell the water to calm down.

I felt the urge to go speak to the young girl, so I went down the steps, and as I watched the power of the wave come in, I was in awe at the older girl swimming, diving under each big wave that came in. Myself, I would not have jumped in. I was afraid. Seeing the power of the ocean, I was afraid for the young girl, but she was fearless. I envied her.

Standing beside the frightened girl, just inches from the edge where swells came up and nearly knocked us off our feet, I stuck my hands out as Spirit guided me.

"When the water is rough and the waves too big, just tell it to calm down," I whispered. Demonstrating what to do, I put my hands out as if I were smoothing out a bedsheet. "Calm down!" I demanded. "Calm down!" I moved my hands as if calming the waters and soon enough, the water was calm. The young girl looked at me as if I had some magical powers.

"How'd you do that?" she asked inquisitively.

Remembering the work of Dr. Emoto, I tried making the description child friendly.

"Well, the water has ears. It listens," I laughed at the revelation. *You already know this,* I heard. Then Spirit or God led me to clap and laugh and sing. Then I heard the voice of God again.

Ask for a big wave.

Laughing and clapping and singing out gratitude to the ocean, I began asking for a big wave to come in. Nothing changed. Looking up at the sky, I was confused.

Now what? I asked Spirit. Then I heard the words.

Feel it.

Confused, I stood there refusing to go up to the edge and feel the water. But then I laughed as I heard the voice again.

Feel it with your heart.

Laughing, I asked the girl what it felt like to jump in. She began telling me how she was sometimes afraid but other times laughing when she jumped in.

"Imagine what it feels like when you are jumping in and laughing," I told her. "Picture it in your mind!" I closed my eyes and pictured the little girl jumping in and laughing with delight. I began clapping again and thanking the ocean for a BIG wave to come in. Sure enough, within seconds the next few waves were bigger than any of the ones before. I even surprised myself. Then Kate came over and joined in and did the same. We talked with the girls a little longer before deciding it was time to head back home.

As Kate drove, I thought about that teachable moment I was given. Water has ears. Our body is made up of water. *Interesting*, I thought. I made a mental note to write when I got home.

It was dark when I arrived back at the house. Cleo and Boy greeted me in the driveway. Boy meowed and rubbed his face against my leg. They were hungry. I fed them their gourmet dinner then headed to the shower. It was a warm night, and I contemplated sleeping out on the lanai. Instead, I slid the patio door to my bedroom wide open. The wind had picked up and cooled off the room. I was tired from all the hiking, so I shut the lights off and fell asleep on top of the covers, snuggled up against Boy.

From a deep slumber, I was suddenly awakened by a sound. I quickly sat up and wiped the sleep from my eyes, trying to adjust to the darkness. Panic struck. An alarm was going off. My first thought was that an intruder had come onto the property, but P had cameras all around. Still, someone could have gotten through the gate. For a moment, I was frozen with fear. I reached for my cell phone and checked the time before turning on the light. Nothing seemed out of place, but the alarm was blaring.

I grabbed the car keys and walked through the house, ready to escape if the need arose. I wasn't sure if I should search the house or get in the car and drive away. P and I never discussed what to do in an emergency. I tiptoed slowly towards the great room, half expecting someone to jump out at me. Turning on all the lights as I went, I headed to the lanai doors. They were open, as they always were, and the cats were sleeping on the patio sofa, undisturbed by the pulsing sound. I noticed then that the alarm wasn't as loud out there. I walked back towards my bedroom, and the sound intensified. I stopped at the closed door next to my room where the noise was coming from.

The door was always closed so I didn't know what was in there. I hadn't been in there before and didn't want to invade P's privacy, but I needed to know what the alarm was.

Slowly, I opened the door, fearful that someone might be in there. It was dark inside, all but a flashing light that appeared to be coming from a desk. I could see a computer but nothing else. I was afraid to turn on the light. I could only see into the room enough to make me unsure of what to do next. I didn't want to know what was in there or what I would find. Knowing was more fearful than not knowing. At least in the dark, a stranger could hide.

I closed the door and walked back to the great room. It was the middle of the night so I couldn't call anyone back home. I thought about calling Kate, but I knew she wouldn't be happy getting a call at this hour. But then I remembered Mary was always up at 3:00 am for work.

I texted Mary.

Call if you're awake. Problem here.

I walked back out to the lanai and called for the kitties to let any intruder know that the house was occupied.

Mary didn't answer. I looked and saw it was 4:44 am. I felt the numbers were a sign from my angels that I would be okay. I remembered reading somewhere that the message meant to be confident about decisions because the angels were with you. I let out a sigh of relief.

"I'm safe," I repeated to myself and let it sink in.

I thought about messaging P, but he was halfway across the world. It seemed silly, so instead, I grabbed my computer and began to write. When I stopped to listen, this time it was to the voice in my own head.

Face your fears or your fears will face you.

I was suddenly reminded of another message I had received from Spirit during a Five Rhythm yoga dance earlier that week. As the dance was winding down, I lay sprawled across the floor when a sudden release of emotions came with the memory of trauma from my early childhood.

I had lost my voice. I was afraid to say no at the time. My whole life had been filled with opportunities for me to find my voice. Abused or abandoned by men since early childhood, learning to find my voice had been a lifelong lesson. I was afraid to voice my opinion, to stand in my own shoes, my own power, and say NO to people. I was afraid because of what I had learned as a child: When you stand up for yourself, you may lose someone you love.

You lost your voice when you were a little girl. Find your voice again.

~

Sitting on the sofa with the alarm still resounding throughout the house, I grabbed a pillow. Clutching it to my chest, I screamed out, "FUCK YOU, FEAR!"

My thoughts turned to P and I wondered why he wasn't checking in on me. There were cameras all over the house and property, so surely, he would have been notified of the alarm.

Finally, I messaged him.

Alarms are going off. I'm scared. What should I do?

No response.

Still frightened, I flipped on the television to have a distraction from the blaring alarms. News stations still had red warning banners scrolling across the bottom of the screen about conflicts with North Korea, so I quickly switched to Netflix. I found a movie and turned up the volume. *Pretty Woman.*

Yes, that would distract me, I thought. Eventually, I fell asleep. It was the rooster that woke me again. It was 5:00 am, and the mysterious alarm had stopped.

I walked around the house and found nothing out of the ordinary. I made coffee and fed Cleo and Boy. Still shaken from the night, I gathered some things and decided to head back to Kate's. Maybe she could explain what had happened or the visions I kept having. I tried calling P but again couldn't get through. I was angry with him for not responding when I needed him. I set food out for the cats and left for the day.

"It does seem odd that he wouldn't return your call and see if you're okay," she agreed after I told her about my night. "Maybe your fear about him leaving you has attracted to you this situation. Maui has a way of testing people." I was still a bit afraid to go back so she invited me to stay for the night.

I was restless all night. I began to contemplate all the possibilities of why an alarm would go off. Everything ran through my imagination from a security alarm that detected an intruder to a bomb that was about to detonate.

The next morning, Kate made us a breakfast of avocado toast and tea, then I told her I was going to head back home to take care of the cats.

"I can't keep running every time I'm afraid," I admitted. "I have to get back to the house. P counts on me to clear out the debris from the pool and to make sure the water pumps go on for the gardens when they're supposed to. I don't want anything to happen to the house while he is gone. Hopefully, he will call today."

"Go up to the market in Paia," she suggested. "Grab some fresh organic veggies to cook yourself a nice dinner tonight. Light some candles, play some music, and tell the house how much you love that it keeps you safe. You know, do a little gratitude ceremony or something."

An hour later, I was standing at the market with an armful of fresh organic produce. As I walked back to the car, I noticed a storefront that advertised shaved ice. Feeling like I deserved a treat, I went in and ordered shaved ice with vanilla ice cream and mango. When I turned to step out of the way for the next customer, I saw the local newspaper sitting on the table beside me. The headline made me gasp.

"Is that for real?" The words shot out of my mouth. "'North Korea Threatens Missile Launches to Hawaii'?" Frantically, I turned the paper all around, looking for a date. The cashier looked at me as if I'd lost my mind.

"Yes, it's a real newspaper," he said. "We get threats all the time. It's no biggie. Besides, that's old news already. It happened the day before yesterday."

It didn't make sense. The day before yesterday was when the alarm went off at the house.

Back in the car, I turned up the music and tried to force all the thoughts from my mind, but they persisted. The little girl within was sure she was smarter than I. She began to taunt me.

P knew Korea was going to send a missile to Hawaii, and that's why he left. He doesn't care about you.

I didn't want to believe that. It felt crazy. Nothing was making any sense. I called Mary, but again there was no answer, no one to help calm me down. I was on my own with two days left until P would be back. Until then, I needed to distract my thoughts with something else.

Just then, Kate called.

"Aloha, Gail Lynn. Did you make it back to P's yet? I just wanted to check in on you."

"I'm still on my way," I said. "I took your advice and stopped in Paia for fresh produce. Did you know that North Korea was threatening to send a missile to Hawaii?"

"No, you know I don't have a television. That's not the kind of stuff I want to fill my head with. It's all programming fear."

"Yeah, I know. Anyways, I'll call you after I get to the house and look around. If you don't hear back from me, give me a call."

When I pulled up the driveway, Boy came out to the car to greet me. He walked with me as I carried the bag of groceries inside. As I got closer to the patio door, I could hear voices. The television was on.

Oh! P must be home early.

I called out for him, but no one answered. No one was there.

Did Cleo or Boy step on the remote? I wondered. I laughed at my justification, but then Cleo jumped up onto the coffee table and sat staring at me. "Was it you?" I asked.

I called Kate to let her know I got home and tell her about the television being turned on.

"I don't know, Gail Lynn. It sounds like you have an intruder coming to the house when you're away. Maybe a local knows when Dr. P leaves and they make use of his house. Didn't you say he goes away for weeks at a time?"

"Yes, he does," I said. "Okay, so tonight, I'll leave all the lights on in the house and turn the music up loud so anyone with an interest in coming here will see the house is occupied. Will you come up and have dinner with me?"

Kate arrived within the hour. We decided to head down to Front Street in Lahaina to do some shopping for a few hours before it got dark.

Walking down the street, I was excited to get to a favorite little gem of a spot I went to for gifts. "There's a cute little boutique across from the Banyan Tree called Maui Memories that I'd like to stop in," I told Kate. "The lady that works there is so kind, and I need to buy a few gifts to bring back to New York."

"Okay, it's just down around the corner from here."

Getting ready to turn the corner, I looked to my left and saw a storefront with its door open. I stopped in my tracks and pointed. "Oh my God!" I exclaimed. I quickly crossed the street paying no attention to Kate. In the doorway stood a figure of a woman who looked as if she were carved out of ice. I stepped closer to get a better look. Circling around the statue, eyeing it up and down, I stopped in front of it and stared in awe at the young woman. Fully naked, she stood with her arms slightly out, palms facing the ocean, and her head tilted back looking to the heavens.

This is me, I whispered.

"Gail Lynn," Kate said, finally catching up. "What's wrong? Why did you come into this studio?"

"Kate, this piece of artwork, look at it. It's me. When I was on Big Island, I hiked through some forests to an open cliff where I stood like this with my face to the sun, feeling like a goddess. It's so bizarre."

"I see you like the work of Michael Wilkinson?" A strange voice intruded into my thoughts. I turned to see a young, dark-haired woman with a pin on her blouse that said, "Sargent's Fine Art."

"Would you like to see more of his work?" she asked.

"Yes! Yes, I would!" I answered.

She led us around the gallery of photos and statues pointing out the other work by the artist. "Do you like any of these?" she asked. Then she gasped, "Wait! There's one more special piece, but it's in the private showing room in the back. Follow me and I'll see if it's available to show you."

Trailing behind her like puppies going to be fed, she stopped in front of a large door, slid it back, and revealed a dark room faintly lit by a small sculpture sitting atop a black velvet pedestal. Intrigued, I slowly entered and walked up to the finely displayed piece of art. I was enamored. Staring at the face of a man about to kiss his beloved, I began to cry.

"Forever," I whispered. "I'll love you forever."

"WHAT?" the curator asked.

"What does this piece of art have to do with Japan and the word, 'forever'?" I asked the woman as tears fell down my cheeks.

"Oh my God," she shrieked as she stood staring at me. Then she quickly turned and shot out of the room leaving us standing there staring after her.

"What's going on, Gail Lynn?" Kate asked. "Why are you crying?" She was just as confused.

"Kate, this is me," I told her. "I did in the arms of my beloved. I was here, in Hawaii, during the attack on Pearl Harbor."

Overcome with emotions as visions passed through my mind, I stepped back to sit on a small leather sofa pushed up against the wall. It wasn't even a minute later when the curator came back into the room waving a paper in her hand. Giving it to me, she stood and gawked at me as if she had seen a ghost.

The paper was a profile of the artist and sculptor, Michael Wilkinson. "He was in the Air Force," the woman said. "He was assigned to Tokyo, Japan. Look on the back of the paper."

I turned the paper over. On the backside was a picture of the acrylic sculpture. It was called, *Forever.*

After an hour of sifting through emotions and visions that kept repeating in my head, I finally decided I needed to purchase the piece of artwork. Before turning to leave, I handed the curator my business card and said, "Please have the artist call me when you speak with him next."

~

Two days later, P was home. He mentioned nothing about my text or call, so I asked if he received my message about the alarms.

"Oh, yes," he said. "I'm sorry. I could not respond. The internet doesn't work well where I was. Besides, the phones get a little crazy when I'm traveling in Iran. Perhaps it was the smoke alarm battery going off." Nothing more was said about it, ever.

The next day P was back to work. August was winding down. Each day I spent hours at the beach now knowing full well it would be ending soon. I took a surf lesson, went horseback riding, and realized my health was the most important thing I had. I sat in the Buddha garden meditating in the mornings and helped P with the gardens after dinner. Nights were filled with marathons of *Star Trek.* Only this time, as soon as I got sleepy, I turned to P, kissed him on the head goodnight, and went to my bedroom to fall asleep.

Then the morning came that I was dreading.

"What day do you want to fly back to New York?" he asked. "I'll go with you and visit my daughter in Buffalo."

I didn't want him to see the disappointment on my face, so I turned my back to him. Having to return to New York was a big disappointment. I didn't want to go back.

"I have to set up my classroom the last week of August," I told him. That evening he booked our flights. We would be leaving in a few days. I went and grabbed my computer and sat out on the lanai to write.

I was healthier and stronger than ever, and I didn't want to go back to the negative environment that had kept me in sickness, pain, and sorrow. I didn't want to face my boss who had ridiculed me in front of my students. I didn't want to hear her shame me for being ill. I began thinking about all the illnesses I had faced over the past few years. Then I thought about what I had been doing on the Big Island and on Maui to heal. I pulled out my computer and began writing great details about my healing journey.

On August 21, we left Maui. Eighteen hours later, we landed in Buffalo. P offered to drive me home, but I declined and told him that my daughter was coming to pick me up. I didn't want him to see my house or the condition it was in. I didn't want him to judge me by the looks of my home, but he insisted and drove me home anyways.

When we pulled up to the house, he stared ahead at it with a blank look on his face. I was embarrassed. A cottage built in 1880, my home looked a little rundown. Old feelings of shame arose in me along with that familiar feeling of not being good enough. He brought my luggage inside and looked around, nodding as he took it all in.

"I bought it last year," I explained. "I remodeled these front two rooms but ran out of money to keep going. So much needs to be repaired still, but I want it to keep the look of the 1800s. The house holds a lot of memories of people who have lived here over the years. I want to honor that." He walked around, nodding, stirring up my inadequacy and shame.

The inner critic took a turn with me, telling me I wasn't good enough for him and that he and his house in Maui were way out of my league. The loose ceiling tiles in the kitchen almost touched his head as he walked through the doorway ducking. I walked back to the front parlor where I stood, defeated. The little girl within me began to cry.

I told you we weren't good enough for him.

"I must go and meet up with my daughter," he said. He reached down for a quick hug and a slight kiss on the cheek. "I'll be in touch."

I wanted to scream, "Please don't go!" but I couldn't manage to get the words out. Instead, I looked into his beautiful eyes fearing I'd never see him again.

"P, you saved my job. You showed me compassion. I found answers to healing. I appreciate you so much."

He smiled and then turned to walk away. "Thank you," he said looking over his shoulder. "I'll be in touch."

I watched from the door as he pulled out of the parking spot and drove away. I stepped back inside and sank to the floor with my head between my legs. The dread of being back in New York descended upon me. The memory of my sickness, pain, and sorrow flooded me. The words "shame" and "unworthiness" were still there in the house, they welcomed me home.

I sat there for a few minutes and looked around the familiar room. What was once my haven now brought me shame. I got myself up, wiped the tears away, and went to the kitchen for a glass of water. There was a pile of mail there that a friend had picked up for me. Right on top was a letter from the school district where I worked.

At least they got their damn doctor's note, I thought.

And I got my health back.

Opening the letter, I was shocked at what I read.

~15~

Stamp of Approval

I read the statement again slowly:

The Board of Education directed you to undergo a medical examination by Dr. Dorfy, an occupational physician, to assess your ability to perform the essential functions of your job as a UPK teacher. Please be advised that if you do not participate in this exam as directed, the District shall withhold your pay.

I felt the old fury rising.

"WHAT?" I screamed. The school was making me go to a DOCTOR'S appointment? For WHAT? I DON'T DO DOCTORS!!

Angry, I called my union representative and read him the letter I had received that directed me to go see their doctor before I was allowed to return to school.

"Yes, Gail, they have that right," the rep said. "And like I told you in June, you have to face the consequences of leaving school before the end of the school let out. And let me give you some advice. It's not just any doctor. They will try to prove you are mentally unstable to teach. You may want to bring someone with you. I've seen this happen before."

"I have an appointment with my own holistic doctor tomorrow. I am having blood work done and everything. Why can't this doctor give me the 'approval' that I'm fit to teach?" I countered.

"Gail, you don't get it. They are trying to find reasons to fire you. If you don't have someone with you taking good notes when you go to the district appointed doctor, the doctor will say you're not fit to teach."

~

The following day, I had a complete blood test panel done. Two days later, I went in for a full checkup.

"Every single one of the tests is normal," the doctor declared. "Better than normal. What have you been doing? These look better than people half your age."

"Hawaii!" I exclaimed. I was on Big Island and Maui all summer. I was happy, stress-free, eating fresh food, sitting in hot springs, dancing, laughing, and I had a near-death experience. AND I found love…I had a magical experience."

"Perhaps I should go there!" the doctor said laughing.

"Okay, but first, can you write me a note for my employer? They are giving me a hard time about returning. I don't know why, but they want a doctor's opinion that I am fit to teach." I couldn't help but laugh. "What do you think? Am I fit to teach?"

"Yes. Most definitely." Grabbing her clipboard, she began to write a return to work note for me. "How old are you? 50? You're healthier than anyone I've seen come through this office in a long time. Kudos to you! A perfect bill of health!"

She handed me the note and wished me well. I turned to walk out with my head held high.

Waving the note high in the air, I sang out. "THE ULTIMATE PRIZE! I WON!! I've got my health back!!"

Walking through the waiting room, ecstatic to have been given the blessing by this doctor that I could return to work, as well as a kudos for taking back my health, people turned to look at me. I simply smiled and waved!

~

I called the HR office and was told that the director did not care about the doctor's note. I had to go to THEIR doctor or else face the consequences. So, a week later, I was heading to Buffalo to see the school appointed doctor for him to determine whether I was *fit* to teach. I asked a friend to attend with me.

Upon entering, the doctor told us he wasn't allowed to provide me with any information from his findings, that his report was strictly for the school.

"Yes," I stated. "So I was told. And that is why I brought my own health advocate. My teacher's union advised me to write down everything that was said in the appointment, so she will be taking notes."

I was very straight forward and matter of fact. I had nothing to hide.

Writing almost verbatim his every question and response, the doctor watched my health advocate vehemently scribbling away. Questioning her need to write everything, my friend told the doctor again, "The teachers union informed Gail to keep a record of all that was discussed in this appointment."

The doctor hesitated, nodded, and continued asking a series of questions all the while watching my health advocate write. He asked about the Lyme disease and when it began. He asked about symptoms and the progression of the disease. Clearly, he was unfamiliar with Lyme disease, and I could see he was being enlightened a bit. I told him about the many misdiagnoses and how doctors had pushed medicine on me rather than try to solve the problem. I told him I stopped using all Western medicine in 2014. I shared my experiences with essential oils as my new wellness tools as well as meditation for stress reduction. He questioned my need to go to Hawaii for healing, and, being completely truthful, he sat back and listened with an open mind. I told him why I went, what I did, and the research I did.

After a brief fifteen minutes, he took a deep breath and looked over at my friend then turned to me.

"You look fine to me and appear fit to teach. That's what will be included in my report to the school. That's all I can share with you. You've got a good head on your shoulders." He turned to look at my friend. "I'm finished here," he said. "You can put away your notes." Then looking back at me, he stuck out his hand as if wanting to handshake a friend. "You are free to leave. Good luck with your school year."

I shook my head. "Of course I'm fit to teach," I said. "The administration just doesn't want me there. I do things a little differently. I believe differently."

I turned and walked out as I heard my friend thank the doctor.

~16~

Integrating Wisdom

I started the school year in September like all the other teachers did, first day jitters and all. It had been quite some time since I had this much energy and excitement to be back teaching again. No accommodations were needed. No part-time days or elevator use. I would not be a "handicap" to my team this year. I would volunteer for everything! I was healthy and strong again. What a relief.

I had been transferred to a new grade level because, as one colleague stated, the district thought I would quit if I had to teach PreK. I let that thought go and was determined to come in each day and be the best damn teacher in the elementary school once again. Remembering the days when both teachers and administrators alike wanted me for their child's teacher, I reveled in the pride that came with that memory.

"I will do it again," I said quietly as I rearranged the furniture in my classroom one day. I took great care in getting my new room ready for the entrance of 18 students; some were still three, but the majority were four-year-olds.

On my first day with students, I stood eagerly at the door greeting parents and students alike. I invited moms and dads to help their child find their coat closet, but for those who came on the bus with no parent, I scooped them up in hugs as tears streamed down their faces. I knew the fear that these little ones were facing. I also knew how to help them overcome it. Right away, we played, we sang songs, and we danced.

Each morning I was given the opportunity to help my little students overcome their fears. I interacted with them at tables building with blocks and dressing dolls and roaring at dinosaurs. As we transitioned to the carpet for our morning circle time, those who needed extra nurturing sat on my lap like my own children used to do. Singing and dancing brought laughter, which helped us all to forget our fears. After the aide set up breakfast at the tables, but before we began eating, I taught the children the importance of gratitude; giving thanks for the helpers in our classroom, for the friends we were making, and for the food that was brought to our room. I was in bliss! I had my life back! AND I was helping young children overcome their fears. I was giving back to life again.

As a colleague passed me in the hallway one morning, I graciously smiled. I knew what was being said. They heard through the rumor mill that the district was going to try to fire me because I left for my healing journey to Hawaii without a doctor's note. But I was ignoring the rumors and sideways glances.

"How do you like PreK, Gail?" a colleague asked one day.

I could tell a fake smile. I could also tell when someone was genuine or not. I responded with honest enthusiasm. "I'm actually loving it! The students are so cute, and we have so much fun singing and dancing every morning!"

The look of surprise made me gloat a little. It didn't matter to me anymore. I had my health back.

~

The honeymoon period lasted about two weeks before the principal began popping into my classroom again. This time though, I wasn't about to be bullied.

I learned I had a voice and I was going to start using it. As she questioned me about best practice, I questioned her right back, including what the law said about student/teacher ratios.

When directed to take my class on a walking field trip across town on a day that thunderstorms were predicted to hit hard, I stood my ground. The other classrooms were still planning to walk the eight blocks across town to visit a fire station. I canceled the trip for my class and told parents that due to the unpredictable storms coming, AND the lack of adult chaperones, I would be making plans for another day. Safety was my priority.

The following morning while I was busy getting my classroom set up for the day, the principal entered and began to reprimand me for not complying.

"You were given a directive to go with the rest of your team on the field trip. Your students should have the same experience as the others." She snarled as she held up the letter I sent home to parents explaining the field trip was being postponed. "You will be written up for insubordination!"

"Look outside. It's going to begin raining soon. Did you see the forecast? AND, just so you know, I just checked with the other teachers, they aren't going today either. Now they are scrambling to get activities set out for when the students arrive this morning. I'm all set, though. Would you like to see my plans?"

I stood there staring at her in disbelief. She didn't care it was about to storm. She didn't care that the other teachers weren't going to walk to the fire station either.

Within the hour, a torrential downpour coupled with thunder and lightning could be seen out the windows. My intuition was right. I was glad I listened to that voice within.

~

A few weeks went by and I began noticing a change in my students. Shortly after breakfast, they became hyperactive and had difficulty sitting listening to a story. Some even became angry. My intuition told me it was the food. I started to pay attention to the labels and counted the sugar content of items brought in for breakfast.

Remembering my own healing journey and the importance of quality food, I questioned "best practice" for the dietary needs of PreK students. Advocating for fresh fruit instead of plastic cups filled with high fructose corn syrup in the canned fruit cocktail, I spoke to the kitchen staff first who had deemed me a troublemaker. I was mocked and told our cafeteria director knows dietary needs better than I would and that, "He doesn't just read some blog, you know."

Next, I brought it to the attention of the principal. Again, I was brushed off. I went above her and called the head administrator of the kitchen stating my concerns about the amount of sugar that is in the breakfast foods for my four-year-old students. Again, I was brushed off. I was disturbed knowing the amount of sugar these students were consuming and how soon after eating they had difficulty focusing.

A big population of our students had difficulty in school. Many were medicated for ADHD, yet no one wanted to do anything about it. I dropped it knowing I had done my part to bring it to the attention of the administrators. I knew if I shared my concerns with parents, I would only fuel the fire of the district's intent to fire me.

Month by month, the tensions became worse. On two different occasions, I got an email stating that the district administration was proceeding with 3020A proceedings, the process a district takes to fire a teacher. Knowing these threats were meant to cause stress or provoke me to react in anger, I tried as hard as I could to ignore them.

In April, I was called into various meetings by different administrators and officials, questioned as to my failure to follow directives by the principal.

When May arrived, each day became more difficult than the last. At times, various staff members would come in and ask me questions only to return to the principal and share what I had said in confidence. It began to be a game I played saying things intentionally to see how fast it got back to the principal. After two of my colleagues offered to help me paint my house only to go back like spies and share my personal information, I vowed to stay away from everyone at the school, beyond my duties, beyond my two best friends, Dar and Deanna.

As I was being left alone with my students more and more, I was put in an awkward position of knowing the state mandates of having two people at all times in the classroom and having to decide how to rectify this situation. Bringing it to the attention of my union did nothing. Bringing it to the attention of the principal did nothing. Calling and speaking to the director of elementary education only led to getting brushed off again.

It was after one of my students got hurt in gym class while the aide was alone, trying to keep all the little ones on task in a game, that I finally decided to call the State Education Department. The more the district refused to care about my students, my aide, and myself, the more I pushed at them to look at best practices and what was really happening in the schools.

I was afraid to give my name for fear of retaliation by the school, but finally, they convinced me. They suggested I speak again with the Director of Elementary Education about the mandates for student/teacher ratios, but I insisted they handle it from there. I was stressed beyond measure. Every single day, an issue arose. More unnecessary "directives" were given to me.

One morning, an email came:

Please call the home of little Johnny and let them know that if he isn't in school every day this week that you will be calling Child Protective Services.

PreK isn't even mandated, I thought. I ignored the email. I knew the family was struggling with the sickness of an older sibling. Stress was mounting as every day I had to go in with compassion for my students yet be prepared for a battle with the administration.

It was mid-May when I arrived at school. Checking my work email, as usual, I opened an email from the teacher's union president:

The district is prepared to go ahead with the 3020A. You may be served with papers today.

I've had two of these emails already since January. How many times are they going to threaten me? Are they trying to put me back in the hospital? I wondered.

My heart began to race, and my chest felt heavy. I sat down and rested my head in my hands. Taking a few deep breaths, I tried to brush off the anger that was rising. My chest began to tighten, and tears threatened. Knowing it would only be another day of harassment, I couldn't take it. I needed to leave.

I called the office and told the secretary I wasn't feeling good and was going to leave to go see my doctor. I asked for someone to come take over my classroom before the children arrived. She sent someone right up. Handing the aid my lesson plan for the day, I left. Thoughts screamed in my head.

I have come too far for these people to put me back in the hospital again! My life is important.

It was getting harder to breathe, so I drove the few blocks to Deanna's house. Frantically pushing the doorbell over and over, the door finally opened, and I fell into her arms crying.

"I can't take this anymore," I sobbed. "They are relentless. Why can't they just leave me alone? They've threatened me again saying they are proceeding with a 3020a meeting to fire me. I did nothing wrong." Rubbing my chest, hoping the pressure would disappear, I followed Deanna as she led me into her living room.

"Sit here," she said. "Calm down. I'll go get you some water." I stuffed my head into the pillow and cried.

"Here, drink some water," she said. "You know Doc Munshi said you're not drinking enough water." She handed me the glass, and I slowly sat up and took a small sip

"My chest hurts, Deanna. I feel like my heart is going to explode out of me. It's hard to breathe. I'm scared."

"What do you mean hurts? Like a pressure or sharp pain? You know what the doctor said about your heart. The Lyme goes into every part of your body. It could be a heart attack."

"No. I'm too young. How do you know the difference between heart attack and anxiety or just being angry? Besides, I was given a clean bill of health in August when I returned from Maui."

"I don't know, but chest pain is serious. If it doesn't get any better, you should have it checked out. What if it's a heart attack?"

"Deanna, please, just sit with me. I can't go to the hospital. They will insist on putting drugs in me and cause more problems. They will end up killing me. They did that to my stepmom. Remember Sheila? They just kept giving her pills until she died. I won't go back to using pharmaceuticals. I can't."

An hour later, my chest was still tight and throbbing. Deanna insisted I go to the hospital, but I didn't want to go. I called another friend, Wendy, who had more experience with this kind of thing and asked her opinion.

"Gail Lynn, this is nothing to take lightly," Wendy asserted. "You get yourself down to that hospital and you tell them how your employer has been causing you all this stress. Stress can lead to heart attacks. Deanna is right."

The old Fear Miser returned in full force. *Could I really be having a heart attack?* I wondered. Like a dry sponge soaking up spilled milk, I soaked up both of their fear.

Upon arrival at the emergency room, Deanna explained to the nurse the stress I was under with my employer and how I left work with chest pains. I was immediately brought in and had my vitals taken. They went through the normal routine, and while the nurse took my blood pressure, I began to get scared.

"I don't take medicine," I informed her. "I don't use pharmaceuticals. I won't put anything foreign into my body." I whimpered, afraid they would start putting needles and drugs in me. "I don't use pharmaceuticals," I repeated.

"Sweetie, you are in good hands," the nurse responded. "Just let me do my job. Heart attacks aren't something to mess with. I want to take you right back and get X-rays and some blood tests started. We need to see what's going on. We'll hook you up to an EKG and a heart monitor to see what's happening."

I began to spew out my spiritual beliefs and how I didn't use medicine in my body. Fighting to keep the nurse from putting an IV in my arm, she finally walked out irritated. Then another nurse came in and calmly explained that no one was putting anything in me. "I just need to take some blood from you so we can get a better understanding of what's happening."

Then another nurse appeared. "The doctor will want to get a read of your cardiac enzymes," she said, "and your white blood cells to see if there's any infection. Then he'll decide what to do."

She pulled out a needle to draw blood.

"Fine," I consented. You can draw blood. But you need the small, baby needle. My veins don't take well to the regular needles. I've had bad experiences with nurses not

288

listening and having to poke me four and five times before having to call a supervisor to get my blood."

The nurse stopped and acknowledged what I had said. "Sounds like you're an old pro," she smiled.

Deanna filled her in about my many trips to the hospital and getting blood draws over the past five years while I battled Lyme disease.

"Hospitals scare her," Deanna said. "And for good reason."

The nurse left with the vials of my blood.

Within 20 minutes, one of the doctors came in with papers in hand to tell me that my cardiac enzymes were elevated.

"You are either going into a heart attack or coming out of a heart attack," he stated. "We need to treat you. I want to run more tests, get a chest X-ray, and I want the nurse to put in an IV in case we need to administer medicine."

My head spun to look at the doctor at the mention of a heart attack. Gripped with fear, I withdrew from the nurse coming at me with a needle.

"WAIT!" I shouted. "I need answers. Do not put that needle in me! I need time to think about this. I need my family here."

Scared that they would kill me, I refused all treatment. Visions of my stepmom replayed in my head. I had tried getting to Phoenix before she passed, but I was too late. The last memory I have of her was of her grabbing the paper cup of pills from the nurse and throwing them across the room shouting, "No!"

My own mind shouted, *Pills kill! Pharmaceuticals kill!*

The doctor was beside himself and left my bedside angrily.

"Gail," Deanna was terrified. "You have to let them treat you. You could die. Let them do their job."

Within a few minutes, my daughter arrived with her boyfriend and a few bottles of essential oils in hand. Looking at me with great concern, Sara reached out for my hand and asked me, "What happened, Mom?"

Unable to control the tears any longer, I finally felt safe. Tears streaming down my face, the words escaped. "Sara, it's the school," I said. "They keep harassing me. My chest hurts. They threatened to fire me again. Now the doctors want to put a needle in me. I can't do it. I won't let them put drugs in me. If I die, it was meant to be, but I can't go back to Western medicine. I've come too far. Please understand," I begged her. "Please don't let them put anything in me. Please just hold my hand. Just love me." I began to sob even harder.

Sara stood, leaned in, and put her arms around me. "I love you, Mom. Everything's going to be okay."

My phone chirped with a text message. Deanna picked it up from the table. "It's Vince. He says, 'Send me healing. I'm having problems with my heart racing.'"

I took the phone from Deanna and texted back.

I'm in ER. Had heart attack. You are feeling me. Please pray.

The doctor came in and questioned who everyone was before continuing. I told him they were family and could hear whatever he had to say.

"You had a mild heart attack and we need to treat you," he said. "I understand you have different religious beliefs and that you won't take any medicine, but at least take an aspirin."

The nurse handed me a paper cup with an aspirin. In my head, I heard my stepmom Sheila loud and clear. "No," I said. "I can't."

I could see the anger rising in his face. "If you won't let us treat you, then why are you here?" The doctor's voice raised an octave and just as he was about to say something more, a nurse popped into the room to let him know he was needed elsewhere. He looked at me with his bushy eyebrows all scrunched together.

"Your cardiac enzymes show you are having a heart attack," he stated. "We need to treat you. We can't just stand by and watch you die."

"How long do I have? Can't you just monitor me? Give me a few hours while I put on some essential oils and pray. I have friends praying for me." The doctor walked out. The nurse came over and said she would give the family time to talk about this. I picked up my phone and texted P hoping he was in Maui and able to receive my message.

I am in the ER having a heart attack.
Could use prayers.

No response came.

~

The nurse kindly took leave so I could be with my family and told me to call for her if I needed anything. Deanna looked over at me with tears in her eyes. "I can't stay," she said, then turned and walked out the door.

Sara leaned in and took my hand. "I love you, Mom. Can't you just–"

"Sara, I love you," I cut her off. "I know I won't die. If it was my time, God would have taken me home when I had my near-death experience in Hawaii last year. I know everything happens for a reason. Perhaps this is my journey, to overcome illness. I met Jesus when I died in Hawaii. He told me that I had to come back to teach. I thought I was supposed to go back to teaching in the school system, but now I know, that's not what he meant. I am to teach what he taught. I am to teach that it is by *faith* we are healed. It is by calling on the power of *love* that we can heal.

"I know that with you sitting here beside me, just loving me like you do, I can help my body heal. My friend, Vince is helping me heal through his prayers and meditation. And when P sees my message, he will send his prayers, too."

Sara just sat there staring at me, tears in her eyes, holding strong like she usually does for me. "I need you," I told her. "I need you to trust me, trust God, whatever God is."

Sara's boyfriend came into the room and over to my bedside. "Your friend said she's sorry," he said, "and I told her don't worry, I'm here!" Sara and I looked at each other and laughed. His lighthearted humor distracted us until Darlene arrived.

"Really, back here again?" she joked. "Haven't you had enough of this place?"

"Thanks for coming, Dar," she gave me a hug. Too tired to laugh, I leaned my head back and asked Sara to explain everything.

I closed my eyes and thought of Bryce. Ho'oponopono came to mind. It had helped heal our relationship, I believed. I closed my eyes and wished him healing and great love then mouthed the words, "I'm sorry, please forgive me, thank you, I love you."

Then I remembered my time on the Big Island with Wendy and all the laughing we did. I thought about P and spending all of August with him in Maui. I thought about the shopping day to get new outfits and about the unconditional love and compassion that he gave me from the moment we met. Then I remembered the feeling of being abandoned when he left me at home in Maui when he went back to Iran. And then the feeling of sadness and abandonment again when he dropped me off at my house in New York. I remembered The Fear Miser.

I'm sorry, please forgive me, thank you, I love you, I prayed Ho'oponopono from my heart. I kept repeating it over and over again in my mind until I heard the voice of God, *Repent, grace, forgiveness, love, gratitude.*

Suddenly I knew everything was going to be okay. I lay there resting with Sara holding my hand. In my mind, I kept telling her I love her. I kept saying I was sorry for failing as a mom.

~

A few hours passed with various nurses checking in on us from time to time. Finally, a nurse walked in with papers in hand and a concerned look on her face. Puzzled, I was almost afraid to ask what the results were.

She took a deep breath and began. "Your cardiac enzymes are back to normal and so are the other blood tests. Everything looks perfect." Shaking her head in disbelief, she held out the report in front of her. "This doesn't make sense."

"Why is that?" I asked.

"Cardiac enzymes should show a gradual decline over time. Yours are normal as if this never happened."

Trying to explain the mystery, I asked, "Is it possible your technician punched in the wrong numbers the first time?"

"No. It's all computer-generated." She stared at me in amazement.

I laughed in celebration. "Do you believe in the power of prayer and meditation, or the power of the mind to heal?" I asked.

She ignored me and turned to address Sara. "Your mom had a mild heart attack. The doctor wants to keep her for observation."

"No, thank you," I chimed in. "My daughter will be able to observe me through the night. I'll stay with her for the next few nights."

Against all the doctor and hospital recommendations, Sara helped me get dressed and we walked out of the hospital, arm in arm, with her boyfriend trailing behind.

A short while later, we were snuggled up on her sofa when I remembered that the lavender and frankincense essential oils got left behind in the hospital room.

"It's okay," I said. "They can have them. Even though you put the frankincense oil on me, it was your love that healed me, Sara."

~

The next day I received a phone call from one of the ER nurses. The head nurse that was on last night had just received new data on some blood work.

"You have *E. Coli*," she said. "You need to get back to the hospital for treatment. It's pretty serious. Left untreated, it can kill you."

I sat staring at the phone for a brief second before shouting. "No," I said. "No, no, no. Why were you checking for *E. Coli*? I don't believe you." I hung up the phone.

Sara's boyfriend looked at me strangely. "Who was that?" he asked.

"Oh," I said, "just someone trying to take my power away."

~17~

Take Back Your Life

The note from the ER physician had me off of work for the remainder of the school year. Summer vacation allowed me to regain my strength, continue learning about energy healing, and practice using the power of the mind for healing. As I continued writing each day, I took time to reflect upon my journey through all the illness. I read, studied, and busied myself with a new adventure.

I began to rent rooms in my house in Lily Dale and named my home "Wishes Fulfilled Retreat" knowing it would be a place where I would help people on their healing journey, where I would help people have their wishes fulfilled. I was making more connections between the Bible, our thoughts, the Laws of the Universe, and our health. I began to make more connections to what caused illnesses and how to heal them.

As summer ended, I received a letter from the school administration. Of course, panic caused my heart to race. But this time, I placed my hand on my heart and began speaking to my body, *It's okay, we will be fine.*

August 28, 2018

To: Gail Lynn

Please be advised that you are being reassigned to District Office to perform duties within your tenure area. Specifically, you have tenure in the district as an elementary education teacher.

You are to report each day no later than 8:00 am. Your attendance by 8:00 am must be confirmed by me or my designee. Report to work ready, willing, and able to work properly and productively- including adhering to all District policies especially pertaining to being under the influence of alcohol or illegal substances. The district will have a workstation for you. You are not to use any personal electronic device to complete district work. The office door should remain open at all times. You are to remain in the office at all times, except to use the lavatory (which you should only use within the District Office) or the break room. You are not to be in any other part of the building. You are assigned a daily lunch from 10:40 am to 11:10 am. You may take your lunch in your assigned office or in the District Office break room. If you choose to leave the grounds for lunch, you must sign out for safety purposes.

Let me remind you that besides what is specifically provided for above, you are prohibited from being on District Property and attending any district activities. Similarly, during the period of your reassignment and leave from your assignment at the school, you should not have contact with any district students or staff concerning this matter, except your union representative. If there is some reason why you feel that you must access District property or attend any District event or activity, you may make a written request to me and your request will be reviewed and considered and either denied or approved. In summary, your restriction on access to school grounds and activities is prohibited unless you receive prior written approval from me as the Superintendent of Schools.

You are further prohibited by Board policy and this directive from engaging in any type of retaliation or having any other individual retaliate against someone on your behalf who you know, believe, or think may be involved in the District's investigation, report of information, or otherwise.

You are hereby advised that your failure to abide by any of the requirements above may result in disciplinary action against you and can be considered insubordination.

The letter fell from my hand floating to the floor. I stood there dumbfounded. *Illegal substances?* I thought. *I don't put anything in my body that isn't natural. And I'm not allowed to talk to staff or students? I'm a teacher! How am I supposed to teach?*

I immediately called the union and inquired about my reassignment. I was informed that all the district was required to do was to keep me in my tenure area. I still had a job, so they were within their limits of what they could do.

Having spoken with two different attorneys and the union attorney, I resolved myself to the idea that I would be doing things like making copies and working on curriculum in the administration offices until I decided what to do next with my life.

I can't keep living my life like this, I thought. *But what am I supposed to do? Rent rooms for $70 or $80 a night in Lily Dale for July and August? What about the rest of the year? How will I support myself? I can't just quit. I am a teacher. I have a pension. I'm supposed to teach until retirement. Will they keep harassing me there until I quit?*

My mind was filled with confusion. "God, where are you?" I whispered as I fell asleep that night.

~

On September 4, 2018, I pulled into the parking lot of the District Administration Office. Not sure what to expect, I entered the school with my purse, cellphone, a notebook, and a pen.

After signing in, a gentleman came through the double doors and said to follow him. He was unfamiliar. I was led down the hallway, past a set of double doors until we reached a room on the right with a label that read "District Storage Room" on the door.

What's this? I wondered.

He walked inside and passed a copy machine to the right of us. Then he pushed open yet another door that was to the left of us. Inside the room, approximately an 8x8 foot area, there was a man sitting at a table with the same manilla folder I had received. Behind him was another man with the same manilla folder on his desk. My escort pointed to an empty desk shoved into the corner.

"You can sit there," he said. "Someone will be down to talk to you later."

I looked at him and then the desk and then back to him again. Confused, I looked around the room. Beige shelving, cold steel, empty.

"You're serious?" I asked.

He lowered his head and left.

I wanted to scream after him, but I stood there in a daze. *I am a teacher! Where are my students?*

The voice inside me asked a million questions. *Why am I in an abandoned storage room?* I wanted to yell, but the other two fellas sat there staring at me.

They looked somewhat familiar, but I wasn't sure what their position was or where they worked. We had a large district with several elementary, middle, and high schools.

There was a laptop on my desk. "Am I supposed to do something here?" I asked them.

"Yeah," one replied. "Sign in with the district name and watch the videos on bloodborne pathogens, sexual harassment, discrimination, and bullying in the workplace."

I opened the computer and signed in. I looked up again at the room full of steel shelves and shivered. It was like a bad dream. *Am I in timeout? What did I do wrong?*

The man behind me with headphones on was watching videos, too. I pushed play and listened to the same videos I had to watch every September, only this time, as I listened to the presentation on discrimination and bullying in the workplace, I was enraged. My thoughts swirled through my mind. My own school administrators had bullied me for several years, and no one cared. No one had done a thing about it.

"These videos are pointless, worthless," I said aloud.

The school had discriminated against me because of my spiritual practices and beliefs and how I used faith healing for years, and they had gotten away with bullying. *This is the perfect picture of hypocrisy*, I thought.

Within the hour, I had completed all the videos. I closed up the laptop and waited for someone to come and tell me what was next. As I sat there, memories popped into my head of being shamed by the principal, of all the times she had harassed me. Then a new vision came to me. *She* felt sad and unworthy and was trying too hard to prove herself. *She* needed love. *She* lacked love in her life.

As much as I didn't want to, I began to feel bad for her. Then Spirit nudged me to do Ho'oponopono. I began to mouth the words saying, "I'm sorry for whatever harm I caused you, whatever sadness I stirred in you. Please forgive me. I never meant you any harm. Thank you. I love you." Still, anger arose in me at her unfair treatment. A single, dense tear cascaded down my cheek. I brushed it away and looked at my phone. It was lunchtime, so I left to sign out.

I drove with no destination in mind and ended up in an Arby's parking lot. Sitting there, I made a phone call to a judge in New York. She had just given a talk at our opening in-service about her own childhood bullies in school. She projected her personal email and phone number on the large screen at the front of the auditorium, and I snapped a picture of it, thinking I may reach out to her and ask for help.

Luckily, she answered my phone call and I quickly explained to her about the storage room where I was sitting all morning.

"Um, hi, um, ...my name is Gail Lynn. I am an elementary school teacher. I ... uh... I was sitting in the school auditorium this morning listening to your talk on bullying. You overcame a lot in your life. And I... I need your help."

"I'm sorry, what was your name?"

"Sorry, it's Gail Lynn. You spoke this morning at the school about bullying. I am being bullied by the administrators at the school. They have taken me out of my classroom and put me in a closet. I need to talk to someone."

The honorable judge apologized and said she didn't have time to talk, her dog was sick, and she needed to call a vet. I felt bad for her dog, but I was also disappointed in her. She just shared her story of being bullied when she was in school and how we should stand up against it, yet she brushed me off.

Hypocrite, I thought. I wished her well and said goodbye.

~

When I got back to school, I ran into a friend. She was happy to see me and asked what I was doing there in the administration office. Trying to keep back the tears, I bit my tongue and pointed to the storage room door sign where I was to enter. She looked confused. I looked around to see if anyone was watching, then I motioned to her to follow me and led her into the storage room.

"That's my workspace," I told her.

Her jaw dropped wide open. She looked at the desk shoved into the corner, then looked back at me, then back to the desk. Her blank stare became glassy.

"You better leave before I get in trouble for showing you," I said. "Keep in touch, friend."

~

The rest of the day I stared at the empty shelves. Tears kept threatening to escape, but I was stronger than that. I took out a pen and paper and began writing the statements for the Hawaiian healing practice, "I'm sorry, please forgive me, thank you, I love you." I wrote and wrote, covering the front page, then turning it over and writing out these statements on the back, and continuing until day one of my new job had ended. It was a very long afternoon.

Day two, September 5, 2018, I arrived on time and sat at the same table pushed up in the corner of the storage room. At 8:15 am, a young woman arrived and told me to follow her. We went upstairs to another storage room. She handed me a paper and told me to organize supplies, and then she left. After an hour I had finished and went back downstairs to my space. I took out paper and wrote a letter to God asking why this was happening to me. I waited for an answer, but my mind was too wrought with sorrow to hear anything from Spirit.

At 10:40 am I left for lunch. Tim Hortons that day. I bought two extra muffins, one for each of the other fellas in purgatory with me. When I got back to the closet, I handed them each a muffin then sat back in my corner and wrote. Visions began to flash in my mind again of another time before this life. When I closed my eyes, I saw the superintendent, only he was dressed in a long brown robe, the kind you see in the Jesus movies. He didn't care for women. He didn't see us as worthy.

I started to cry and was glad I was facing the wall. I sat and prayed and allowed the tears to gently fall until quitting time.

Day three. At 8:15 am I sat and wrote letters to God again. I went to the bathroom and had a hard cry. I spent the day working on my manuscript, staring at the walls, and meditating. I went for lunch, came back, then sat and cried for the rest of the afternoon.

Day four. By 8:25 am I was angry and sad, crying with snot running from my nose. I didn't have a tissue but didn't want the other guys to see me like this. I put my head on the desk and watched the drops fall from my face to the floor. At lunchtime I let them leave first. After the break, I worked on my manuscript. At some point, I knew I was done. Done with being treated like I didn't matter. I decided to turn in my keys the next day.

Day five, September 7, 2018. At 8:15 am, I quit. I wrote a note to my oppressors:

> I'm done, I'm done, I'm done. You will not confine me any longer. I matter. I am important. My health matters. You will never bully me again. You win for now, but in the end, God wins. Light always trumps darkness. Jesus himself said, "For I know the plans I have for you, plans to prosper you, not to harm you. Dear Jesus, make this right."

I left for lunch and returned with renewed strength.

As I continued writing my story, a young administrator entered the room and sat down next to me. She looked me in the eyes and as she began to talk, tears fell down my cheeks. I hated that I was crying, but this time it was not out of weakness but out of happiness. I was ready to take back my life.

"I'm sorry for all this," she said. Seeing the tears, she looked away, uncomfortable. "I don't know what's going on, but maybe next week will be better. If I can do anything to help, please –"

"There won't be a next week," I put my keys on the table. "I quit."

She didn't know what to say. Now the tears formed in her eyes, and I almost felt bad for her.

"You work for adults who hurt their employees," I choked out the words. "I will pray for you. Look at this room. No one should be treated this way. I did nothing wrong. All I wanted was to heal. I wanted to overcome the years of sickness and pain. And I did it. Even though it has cost me my job, I would do it again, because I finally realized something. I matter. I am important."

She sat for a moment then reached out to hug me and said, "I wish you all the best, Gail Lynn." She picked up the keys and walked out.

The clock read 2:22 pm. I thought of my friend, Mary.

What would Mary do? I asked myself.

Then Mary of Magdala appeared in my mind, the woman in history whose story had been hidden for so long, the woman who had been shamed and shunned.

I am you. We are One, I heard her whisper in my heart.

I packed up my personal belongings and left. Walking with my head held high, I sang Ho'oponopono on my way out the door.

"I'm sorry, please forgive me, I thank you, and I love you! I'm sorry, please forgive me, I thank you, and I love, love, love, you!"

~

Later that evening, I called each of my children to tell them the news. "Mom quit!" I said proudly.

They weren't as enthused as I was. They worried about me finding another job, and I so I told them, "I don't know what I am going to do right now, but I matter, and that's all that counts."

The next day I called the union president and explained the situation. I was told, basically, that I should be happy I had a job. "You left two days before school was out," said the president. "I told you that you'd have consequences."

I asked for the phone number of the union lawyer who represented teachers. Speaking to him, I didn't feel any better. "My job was to make sure you had a job. And you did, you did have a job. If you want, we could try to seek some type of settlement, but it would be highly unlikely that the district would go for that."

I spent the weekend alone grieving and contemplating the experience in the storage room and trying to make sense of something so completely heart-wrenching. Sitting in the quiet, contemplating my life and talking with myself and God, I heard the voice.

The Laws of Nature are always just.

The weekend passed, and when Monday arrived, my heart felt such sadness. Luckily for me, my daughter asked me to come over and help her and her boyfriend. They needed to get a guest list together for their wedding. Her boyfriend had proposed over the summer. We had to organize a wedding in ten weeks before he left for basic training.

I began to realize it was a blessing not to have to go to work. I felt blessed to be home and able to be with my daughter each day. As October arrived, we were less than a month away from the big day. Everything came together so easily, and I was grateful that I had every day free to meet with florists and caterers and to visit different venues.

My phone rang one morning. The name on the screen set my heart racing.

"P!" I was so happy to hear from him. We hadn't talked in months. "How are you? It's so good to hear from you!"

"Good morning," he said in his usual manner. "I'm good. How are you?"

"Wow! I'm good, thank you. And *really* good, now that I talk to you! What's new? Where are you? What have you been up to?"

P laughed at my onslaught of questions. He was in Buffalo visiting his daughter and wanted to know if I was free for dinner that night

"Yes!" I exclaimed. "Yes, of course I'm free!"

"Good. How's 6 o'clock? I'll come pick you up, and you can lead us to a local place for a bite to eat."

"That sounds perfect," I exhaled. "It's so good to hear from you, P."

I spent the next several hours going through my closet deciding what to wear, like a teenager getting ready for prom. I set out my clothes, jewelry, and shoes, then called Mary. She didn't answer, so I left a message.

"Guess who's coming to see me tonight!" I sang into her voicemail.

I made a quick trip to the store for some fresh flowers, put music on as I showered, and readied myself to see P. As the time drew nearer, I kept checking out the window like an eager teenager waiting for my date to arrive. When he finally pulled up, my heart pitter-pattered with excitement. He looked as handsome as ever. His tall, thin frame was dressed in tailored slacks with a sage green shirt that matched his big, beautiful eyes. His lips curled up into a slight smile. The sight of him brought back many beautiful memories.

"You look beautiful," he said leaning in for a warm embrace. My heart felt full as I held onto him, wanting to linger a little longer.

"You look *and* smell good," I smiled. "How are you these days? Sit, tell me what's new with you."

As he told me about his travels, I pictured in my mind all the lovely places he had experienced. In awe and wonder, I loved his sense of adventure.

"Tell me about you," he said. "What's new?"

As I contemplated where to begin, a million thoughts raced through my mind. Disheartened and angry at the memory of being put in a storage room, I began to explain.

"Well, I quit my job. I'm not sure what I'm doing now other than helping my daughter plan her wedding. Other than that, I'm not sure what I'm supposed to do with my life."

"Well, why not come home with me?"

My heart leaped. I was without words to respond.

"My plane leaves at 5:00 am. I fly out of Toronto."

"What? You're leaving already, P?"

"Yes. Tonight. I need to head to Toronto to return my car and get through customs. I fly back home to Maui in the morning."

I stared at him to see if he was joking or serious. I couldn't tell by his smile.

"Grab your computer," he continued. "Pull up flights and we'll see if you can get a flight out in the morning as well. We can coordinate our itineraries, maybe get on the same flight."

"You're serious? P, I can't just fly out tomorrow!"

"Why not?"

"My daughter is getting married in a few weeks. I need to be here for her."

"What's left to do this week? Come for ten days, then fly back here for the wedding, and then after the wedding is over, come back home to Maui?"

I was thrilled. Maui did feel like home. He had no idea what I had been through the last couple of months, but I knew then that my angels were watching over me. They knew I needed him.

I pulled out my computer and handed it over to P. "You're the expert," I laughed. Within minutes he found me a flight, took out his credit card, and booked my trip. Then closing my laptop, he handed it back, smiling.

"You better get packing."

I hugged him, hard.

I was going home.

~Epilogue~

Love's Potential

Those ten days that I spent with P in Maui were some of the happiest days of my life. He finally agreed to hike with me up the western Maui mountains. We drove the Road to Hana and hiked several waterfalls and then stopped for roadside chicken barbeque. At the halfway marker, we bought three coconuts from a local to bring home. We planted them in the gardens and named them, Coco 1, Coco 2, and Coco 3.

We fell asleep on the sofa each night, side by side, wrapped up in each other's arms again. This time, I could tell, P needed the love and companionship just as much as I did. The first few days were filled with *Star Trek* episodes. He would point out little bits of foreshadowing that had appeared years later in real life.

We spent hours caring for the gardens, the kitties, and exploring. Cleo and Boy were happy to have me back home and followed me everywhere. Then one afternoon, I even talked P into going to the beach with me. I was overcome with joy when I saw him smile at the water as a turtle swam by and brushed up against his leg. I was a little nervous at how close they came until he reminded me that turtles feel our joy and want to play with us. *Joy*, I thought. *This is what joy feels like!*

There is no heaven in the sky, I heard the voice of God in my mind say to me. *This here is heaven. Heaven is a state of mind.*

~

As my daughter's big wedding day approached, I asked P to join me as my date. That's when things changed again between us. He said he had plans to fly back to Iran again to visit with his family. He was finally getting the opportunity to get to know some of his relatives and the Persian culture in Iran, and he had met a young woman while traveling the Middle East with his family over the winter.

Wondering who the woman was and what she meant to him, I asked.

"She's Persian," he explained. "She's my companion during the weeks when I'm in Iran." That's all that was said.

He shared his joy of getting to know the Persian culture better, the Persian people. "It has been years since I've been there," he said. He told me stories of how they were lovely, kind, compassionate, people who were willing to take others in off the street if they were hungry.

Just like P, I thought.

Now, P and I, our story, had a new character in it. What was once a potential for love between us was now over. He had a potential for love in Iran. I could feel his joy when he talked about the culture and his family there. I found joy being in Maui, and I have come to understand the importance of being happy. I was glad to see that he found joy, too. I was happy to see the smile on his face, even though it wasn't about me.

And that's when I realized something had really shifted in me. Love...true love...is unconditional. Love isn't about me. It's about the other person.

I love P, I thought to myself. *I would have done just about anything to see him happy, to help him get healthy and feel joy again.* And then I thought about Bryce and when I saw him with the new girl on that Fourth of July so many years ago. I should have blessed him and been happy for him, just like I was happy for P. I was naïve and foolish and said hurtful words to Bryce. Saying he had a disease brought disease back to me. I just knew. It's universal law. Cause and effect.

Being claircognizant, there are some things you just cannot explain.

~

I flew back to New York for three weeks and spent all of my time with my daughter finalizing plans for her wedding day. Seeing my daughter so in love made me the happiest mom ever. All through the wedding, I watched as my three children danced, laughed, and carried on with the loves of their lives. Looking at my son Josh gazing into the eyes of his date for the night, I could see a spark that had been missing for a long time. *She's the one*, my higher self said. I just knew.

When I finally got home and turned back the covers to climb into bed, I grabbed my journal. Missing P, I began paging through the entries of the previous year skimming through January and February, slowing down to read each entry in March, I began to notice something. Then April, May, and June were more of the same. I was writing each journal entry, "Dear Soul Mate…"

Then I re-read the last entry before meeting P on June 17, 2017, right before I got on the plane in Buffalo, New York when my life changed forever.

June 17, 2017
Good morning my love, only a few more days! I can't wait to be in your arms, hold you, touch you, kiss

311

you, love you. I am so in love with you. I am so in love with us, I am so in love with life! We will continue to create beautiful memories together as we share our daily life! I see us holding hands on walks, I see us cooking together and sharing meals, long conversations, books, food, life, the divine spark, and love. Have a beautiful day!

(that evening) ...My beloved, my heart longs to be in your arms again, legs intertwined as we sleep holding each other with deep love. Thank you for being my rock, my comfort, my supporter. Rest well my love, feel my longing my love.

June 18, 2017
Good morning my love. I am going to see Momma today. Can you send her your blessings of love? Can you please ask her to stay until she has the chance to meet you? I want her to be here to see us together in beautiful bliss and allow her to experience our love together. Thank you, my love, thank you, until we are together, days, hours moments away, know my love for you runs so deep, always.

(that evening) ...Thank you, my love.

June 19, 2017
Good morning my love, thank you for keeping me close to your heart all night. Momma is doing much better and I am pleased. Continue to pray with me for a miracle in her healing. Help me to take her on a trip that is magical. I love you Jesus. I love you Creator. I love you boyfriend, life partner, fiancé, spouse, life-long lover. Thank you for joining me in these next 50 years.

Always, I love you!

(that evening) ... Goodnight my love, hold me tight.

June 20, 2017
My love for you continues to grow stronger each day!

June 21, 2017
I am going to Hawaii to heal, to grow, to evolve, to learn to prosper, to love to make a difference in our World. I will flourish. I will step into greater prosperity. I will have greater wealth and greater health abundantly, greater than I ever could have imagined. I see my life happy, healthy, and financially successful. I see so much money flowing into my life in a never-ending stream. Wealthy and healthy is my birthright and I claim that NOW. I call upon all my loved ones, I call upon the angels, Archangel Michael, and the Mighty legion of protectors and I call upon the Christ light within to fill me, protect me, and guide me. I ask that you help me in these decisions and knowing undoubtedly the next step. Lift me in love. I ask these things and step into faith that it is so. God is with me, God is in me. Thank you, thank, you, thank you. I love you.

June 22, 2017
MAUI BOUND!

~

I shot upright and my mouth fell open. I wrote about a soul mate. I wrote *to* a soul mate, about falling asleep side by side on the sofa, about watching movies and our feet intertwined. Did I *create* P? Did I write my own love story?
Oh P, where are you now? Are you in Iran and in love?

~

Perhaps Bryce and P and all the others were meant to be a training course for the best love story ever told. Perhaps all the characters in my story were put there, in the perfect place, to help me learn lessons in love.

I am excited about the prospect of love in my life again! I know that there is a divine presence that hears me, sees me, and knows my heart. This presence, whether you call it God, Spirit, Creator, Allah, Jehovah, or field of energy; it prepares us all to open our hearts to love.

The greatest love story ever told is coming! I know it is on the way. I just DO! It's on the horizon. It's what the journey is about. Love is what heals all that ails us. It is the medicine that has the potential to cure any disease. I received it. I felt it. I healed.

I matter and you matter, too.

Oh, Reader, have you come to realize that yet? Have you come to see your own place on the hero/heroine's journey? Take a look at your life and the character role each person has. See them through new eyes. Forgive them for any mistakes they have made. Secret teachings include the verse, "Forgive others as you have been forgiven."

Watch your life begin to shift as you lead with love.

~

THE GREATEST COMMANDMENT is to LOVE the Lord your God with all your heart, with all your soul, with all your mind...And since the Kingdom of God is within you, this means...LOVE YOURSELF!

THEN, love others as yourself...

That's what heroines do!

~Questions for Self-Reflection~

What do I know about my parents' lives?

What happened between birth and age five?

What do I remember about my elementary school years?

High school years?

How did college life affect me?

Who are the influential characters in my life?

What trauma have I endured and how did I react?

Who do I need to forgive?

Who do I need to ask for forgiveness?

Think of someone who has hurt you. They are a mirror for something you caused in another. Repeat the phrases of Ho'oponopono: I'm sorry, please forgive me, thank you, I love you. But only if you really mean it.

Acknowledgments

To Dr. P, my Earth angel. You gave me heaven on Earth. I'm forever grateful. I love you unconditionally.

To my editor, and Artemis, thank you for helping me to see this through.

To all my loved ones in the spirit world, thank you for leading me home to love.

To all the "villains" in my story, you played your role well. Thank you for choosing the tough characters.

To Grandma Brumagin and Sheila, since the beginning of writing this book, your presence wrapped me in love, reminding me that I DO matter. Thank you.

To all of you known or unknown to me, who pick up this book, who have those thoughts no matter how fleeting that, "I'm not good enough. I can't do this life. I'm just too tired to continue" … please hear my words, you ARE good enough. YOU! No matter what has happened in the past, no matter what your present circumstances, YOU matter, your life matters, and you CAN take back your life and live it joyfully! No matter what illness you may have, no matter what your struggle, you can find your way out to living a better life with greater love!

To the late Wayne Dyer, your teachings, your light, your Divine love, and your wisdom all changed my life forever. I love you. Thank you for being with me on that airplane! Thank you for sending me the doctor I needed at the perfect time!

To the late Shirley Calkins Smith, Lily Dale Medium, friend, lover of life, the one who gave me strength and understanding of what it is to be a woman empowered.

Women's Empowerment Weekend, Lily Dale June 4-5, 2012. I AM an empowered woman!

To Tom Rugani and my healing sisters, Lorraine, Jean, Jewell, and Brenda. I will always hold dear to me the healing in our gatherings. I love you as my sisters.

To Judith Rochester, for your unconditional love and support, for believing in me and giving me the courage to write my story.

To Deanna and Darlene, for all the times you held my hand and stripped me naked in the Emergency Room, I love you. I am so grateful for you. To Steve M., thank you for making a difference in my life. Yes, I matter!

To Wendy, Laurie, and Denise…to Boob, Judy, Janelle, Vince, Scott, Jacob, Glenn, Jenn P., Lisa W., Lisa R., Jen V., Jeanne, Kelly, Robin, Jen N., and to all of you too numerous to mention who shared moments with me, who prayed, laughed, cried, snuggled, rubbed my feet or danced in my living room, I am grateful for your love. May you continue to love everyone bigger, deeper, unconditionally. Our world needs more love.

To Mary O'Donnell, thank you for being there to push me to keep going. Your never-ending support kept me moving forward through all the times when I questioned my worth.

To Bryce, for all the years we tried to get love right. I wish you sweet love that fills you completely and heals all wounds. I love you unconditionally. Don't go far, XOX.

To my first "ex," we were so young and didn't know any better, but we have two beautiful men who are still learning how to love. Thank you.

To my second "ex," I'm sorry. You are a kind, loving, human being and a wonderful father to our *three* children.

To attorney JJ, I am grateful for you. Thank you for standing for the underdogs. Always remember, it is done, as you BELIEVE; the greater your faith, the greater the mountain that you will move. Blessings to you and to all your future clients.

To all my past students… teaching and inspiring you was my world. Pushing you to be better every day was my way of saying, "I see greatness in you! You can do anything and overcome anything as long as you believe in yourself!"

To my siblings, Anne, Tom, and Darrin, thank you for choosing me to be your sister in this lifetime. You have endured so much, and I am proud of you. I love you always, unconditionally. I wish you greater love, happiness, health, and success.

To my father, the immigrant from Sicily, I finally understand. I love you no matter what. You will always be my daddy. And to my momma, I'm sorry you had so many years of sadness. I pray next time around you have an abundance of great health, wealth, and happiness. Thank you for always lending a shoulder to cry on, I love you more!

To Alycia, KK, Caden, Kate and Al, Big Jim, Seth, Melissa … and my extended family, you are all magnificent!

And lastly, to my children, there are no words to describe the depths of my love for you. I do not know how to even begin to explain our lives together, but maybe my story will help you. I'm sorry for all the mistakes I made. I fell short of being the ideal mom, but I did the best I knew how. Thank you for loving me through it all. Always remember, you are more powerful than you know. I'll always be here to support you and cheer you on as you follow your own path. You have the power within you to have, be, and do anything you want! YOU are the CREATOR of your own life. Picture it the way you want and go after it. "The force is with you!" It's in your heart. See everything that you do in life, be a success. YOU co-create your life with every thought you have and every word you speak. May all your dreams come true. I love you always. ~Mom

Appendix

A. *Lyme Disease – The Basics.* The York Lyme Disease Support Group. www.yorkpalyme.org

LYME DISEASE SYMPTOM CHECKLIST

The following are symptoms associated with Lyme and tick-borne co-infections.
Not all cases are caused by a tick bite, and the "bull's eye" rash occurs in less than 50% of the cases.

Since Lyme Disease tests are only 40% accurate, the majority of cases are "negative."

Musculoskeletal System
• Joint pain or swelling
• Stiffness of joints, back or neck
• Movement of pain or swelling to different joints
• Creaking, popping, cracking joints
• Muscle pain or cramps
• General Muscle Pain/Tenderness (fibromyalgia)
• Hand stiffness
• Foot pain (aches or burning)
• Bone sensitivity, esp. the spine
• Clumsiness
• Backache
• Rib soreness
• Tendonitis
• Gait disturbance

Neurologic System

- Headache (persistent / intermittent / severe / migraine-like)
- Bell's Palsy (facial paralysis)
- Burning, stabbing, or shooting pains
- Tremors or unexplained shaking
- Numbness in parts of body / extremities
- Tingling sensations (crawling on skin)
- Weakness or partial paralysis
- Lightheadedness, wooziness, fainting
- Twitching of muscles
- Poor balance, dizziness, difficulty walking
- Increased motion sickness
- Alternating warm / cool sensations
- Constant low body temperature
- Stroke symptoms, seizures
- Taste / smell abnormalities
- Abnormal blood flow in brain
- Diminished reflexes
- Hearing music or sounds others can't hear
- Visual, auditory or odor hallucinations
- Restless legs or periodic limb movement disorder

Psychological Well-being
- Mood swings, irritability
- Easily frustrated
- Unusual depression
- Crying impulses for no reason
- Over-emotional reactions, crying easily
- Panic or anxiety attacks
- Rage, aggression
- Insomnia (difficulty falling or staying asleep), sleep apnea, narcolepsy
- Disturbed sleep: too much, too little, fractionated, early awakening
- Nightmares
- Paranoia
- Suicidal thoughts
- Obsessive-compulsive behaviors

- Disorientation (getting or feeling lost)
- Depersonalization (losing touch with reality, feeling "unreal")
- Low self-esteem
- Bitterness, guilt, alienation
- Bipolar, psychosis-like disorder

Mental Capabilities
- Memory loss (short or long term)
- Distorted memory
- Confusion, difficulty in thinking
- Difficulty with focus, concentration, reading ("Brain fog")
- Inattention
- Forgetting how to perform simple tasks
- Speech difficulty (slurred, slow, hesitant)
- Word finding trouble
- Forgetfulness
- Letter, number, word reversals
- Stammering, stuttering speech
- Going to wrong places
- Getting lost in familiar places

Eyes, Vision
- Floaters
- Double or blurry vision
- Eye pain, pressure in eyes
- Light sensitivity
- Tearing eyes, dry eyes
- Vision loss, Blindness
- Swelling around eyes
- Flashing lights

Ears, Hearing
- Decreased hearing in one or both ears
- Buzzing, clicking, or ringing
- Sound sensitivity
- Pain in ears

Digestive and Excretory System
- Diarrhea / Constipation
- Abdominal pain / Bloating
- Irritable bladder (trouble starting, stopping)
- Frequent need to urinate
- Upset stomach, vomiting
- Gastroesophageal reflux (acid reflux or GERD)
- Anorexia

Respiratory / Circulatory System
- Shortness of breath
- Chest pain
- Night sweats / Unexplained chills
- Heart palpitations, extra beats, pulse skips
- Heart block / Heart attack
- Heart murmurs / Valve prolapse
- Elevated or low blood pressure
- Frequent and easy bruising of skin
- Cough (odd, unexplained)

Reproduction
- Loss of sex drive
- Sexual dysfunction
- Unexplained menstrual pain, irregularity
- Unexplained breast/nipple pain, discharge
- Testicular or pelvic pain

Head, Face, Neck
- Neck stiffness, pain, creaks, cracks
- Twitching of facial or other muscles
- Painful teeth or gums
- Difficulty swallowing
- Sore throat
- Unexplained hair loss
- Scalp rash
- Hoarseness, drippy nose (unexplained)

General Well-being
- Extreme, persistent fatigue, poor stamina
- Symptoms change, come and go
- Pain moves to different body parts
- Unexplained weight gain or loss
- Malaise
- Any type of rash / Itching
- Night sweats (drenching)
- Unexplained sweating
- Swollen glands
- Unexplained fevers (high or low)
- Continual infections (sinus, kidney, yeast, bladder)
- Increased sensitivity to allergens
- Exaggerated response to alcohol or sugar
- Sugar craving
- Nodules under the skin
- Experience of flu-like symptoms, and have not felt well since

Common Misdiagnoses
- Multiple Sclerosis
- Parkinson's Disease
- Lupus, Gout, Hepatitis
- Carpal Tunnel Syndrome
- Meniere's disease / TMJ (jaw pain)
- Fibromyalgia
- Rheumatoid Arthritis
- Chronic Fatigue Syndrome
- ALS (Lou Gehrig's Disease)
- Crohn's Disease
- Psychological/psychiatric symptoms
- ADHD (Attention Deficit Hyperactivity Disorder)
- Epstein-Barr virus infection

B. Writing from my students

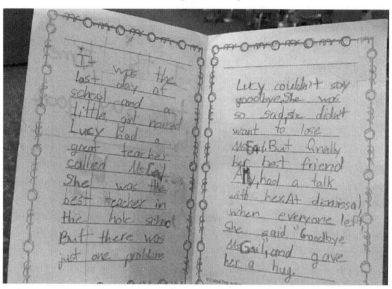

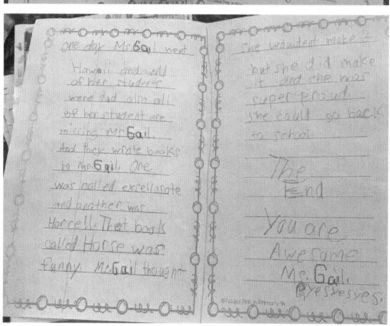

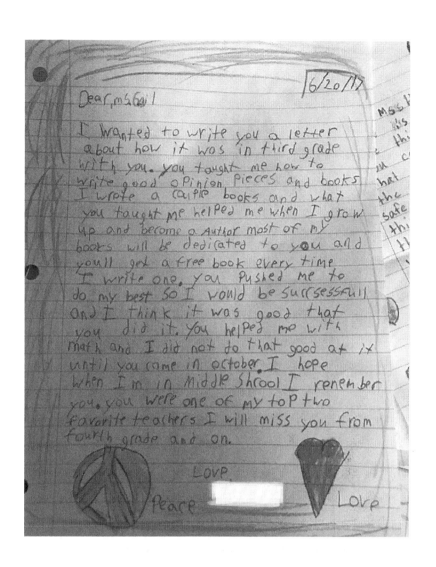

Dear, ms Gail

I wanted to write you a letter
about how it was in third grade
with you. you taught me how to
write good opinion pieces and books
I wrote a couple books and what
you taught me helped me when I grow
up and become a Author most of my
books will be dedicated to you and
you'll get a free book every time
I write one. you pushed me to
do my best so I would be successfull
and I think it was good that
you did it. You helped me with
math and I did not do that good at it
until you came in october. I hope
when I'm in middle shrool I remember
you. you were one of my top two
favorite teachers I will miss you from
fourth grade and on.

LOVE.

Peace   LOVE

327

happy last day
of school miss Gail
Dear: Miss Gail

I thank you
for being my
third grad teacher
and when you
first cam thow
that door I
jumped right
out of my
chare saying
miss Gail!
and sens that
verg last I'v
gave you love
and kindnes
and when you
sed that it
was your
last day today
I'll give you as
many hugs as
you want
miss Gail.

Love
Miss
Gail
frome.

C. Journal entry

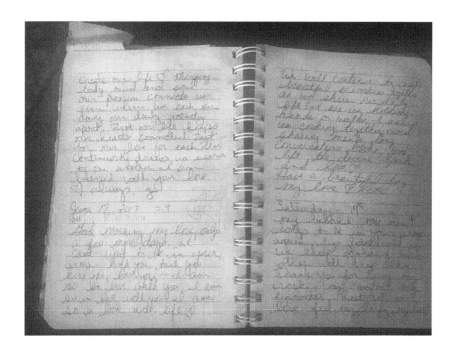

D. Michael Wilkinson's sculptures, *Lodestar* and *Forever*

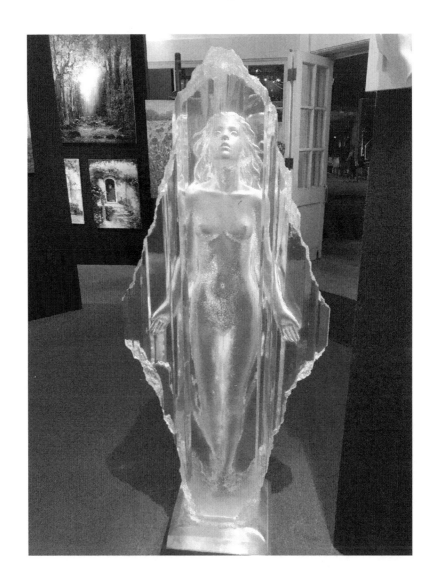

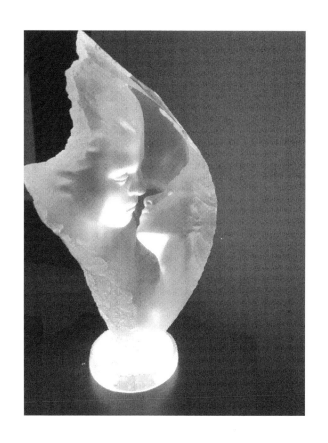

E. Storage room office and desk

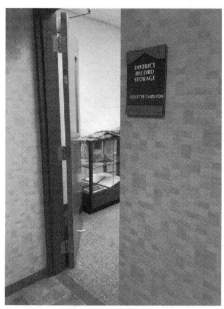

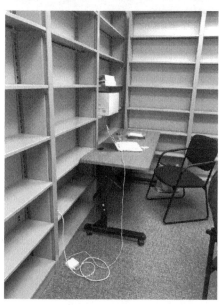

F. List of Influential Books

Beckwith, Michael Bernard. *Life Visioning (16pt Large Print Edition)*. ReadHowYouWant, 2012.

Braden, Gregg. *Spontaneous Healing of Belief - Shattering the Paradigm of False Limits*. Hay House Inc, 2008.

Brown, Brene. *Gifts of Imperfection*. Vermilion, 2020.

Byrne, Rhonda. *The Secret*. Atria Books, 2018.

Campbell, Joseph. *The Power of Myth / Joseph Campbell*. Doubleday, 1988.

Dyer, Wayne W. *Change Your Thoughts - Change Your Life: Living the Wisdom of the Tao*. Hay House, 2013.

Dyer, Wayne W. *Living the Wisdom of the Tao*. Hay House, 2016.

Dyer, Wayne W. *The Power of Intention: Learning to Co-Create Your World Your Way*. Hay House, Inc., 2010.

Dyer, Wayne W. *Wishes Fulfilled: Mastering the Art of Manifesting*. Hay House, 2013.

Emoto, Masaru, and Elizabeth Puttick. *The Healing Power of Water*. Hay House, Inc., 2007.

Emoto, Masaru. *The Secret of Water*. Simon & Schuster, 2006.

Fox, Emmet. *Power Through Constructive Thinking*. HarperCollins e-Books, 2010.

Goddard, Neville. *Your Faith is Your Fortune*. Bibliotech Press, 2019.

Goldman, Jonathan. *The Divine Name: the Sound That Can Change the World*. Hay House, 2010.

Haanel, Charles F. *The Master Key System*. Dover Publications, 2018.

Hay, Louise L./ Schulz, Mona Lisa. *All Is Well: Heal Your Body With Medicine, Affirmations, and Intuition*. Hay House Inc, 2014.

Hay, Louise L. *You Can Heal Your Life*. Hay House, Inc., 2017.

Hesse, Hermann. *Siddhartha - Hermann Hesse*. Spark Publishing, 2005.

Hicks, Esther. *Getting into the Vortex!: the Law of Attraction in Action*. Hay House Inc, 2010.

Hicks, Jerry. *The Astonishing Power of Emotion*. Hay House Inc, 2020.

Holmes, Ernest. *The Hidden Power of the Bible: What Science of Mind Reveals about the Bible and You: Originally Published as The Bible in the Light of Religious Science*. J.P. Tarcher/Penguin, 2006.

Holmes, Ernest. *The Science of Mind: the Complete Edition*. Jeremy P. Tarcher, 2010.

Jung, Carl Gustav., and Robert Coles. *Selected Writings: Carl Gustav Jung*. Book-of-the-Month Club, 1997.

King, Deborah. *Be Your Own Shaman: Heal Yourself and Others with 21st-Century Energy Medicine*. Hay House, 2012.

King, Deborah. *Truth Heals: What You Can Hide Can Hurt You*. Hay House, 2009.

King, Serge. *Huna: Ancient Hawaiian Secrets for Modern Living*. Atria Books, 2008.

King, Serge Kahili. *Urban Shaman*. Touchstone, 1990.

Lipton, Bruce H. *The Biology of Belief*. Spirit 2000, Inc., 2003.

McTaggart, Lynne. *The Intention Experiment: Using Your Thoughts to Change Your Life and the World*. Atria Paperback, 2013.

Morse, Robert. *The Detox Miracle Source Book*. Kalindi Press, 2004.

Ober, Clinton, et al. *Earthing: the Most Important Health Discovery Ever?* Read How You Want, 2014.

Radin, Dean I. *Real Magic*. Harmony, 2018.

Radin, Dean I. *The Conscious Universe: the Scientific Truth of Psychic Phenomena*. HarperOne, 2009.

Redfield, James. *The Celestine Prophecy*. Random House Australia, 2011.

Shinn, Florence Scovel. *The Game of Life, and Other Works*. Lushena Books, 2001.

Shook, E. Victoria. *Ho'oponopono: Contemporary Uses of a Hawaiian Problem-Solving Process*. Univ. of Hawai'i Pr., 1995.

Tolle, Eckert. *The Power of Now*. New World Library, 2004.

Walsch, Neale Donald. *Conversations with God: an Uncommon Dialogue*. Hampton Roads Publishing Company, 1997.

Williamson, Marianne. *A Return to Love: Reflections on the Principles of a Course in Miracles*. Thorsons Classics, 2015.

Yogananda, and Kriyananda. *The Essence of Self-Realization: the Wisdom of Paramhansa Yogananda*. Crystal Clarity Publishers, 2010.

G. Influential Documentaries

Finding Joe. Directed by Patrick Takaya Solomon, Balcony Releasing *and* Pat and Pat Productions, 2011.

Heal. Directed by Kelly Noonan, Elevative Entertainment *and* i2i Productions, 2017.

Under Our Skin. Directed by Andrew Abrahams Wilson, Open Eye Pictures, 2008.

About The Author

Gail Lynn is an Ordained Minister, Life Coach, Intuitive, Energy Healer, spiritual teacher, retreat leader, speaker, and best-selling author. She has traveled across the US and Canada, delivering keynote addresses and motivational speeches, and sharing insights on the practice of love and forgiveness to heal old patterns and take back your life.

If you need guidance as you develop your own life map, connect with her at www.gail-lynn.com, or in the world-renowned spiritual community of Lily Dale, NY, where she runs her business, Wishes Fulfilled Retreat. Look for her next book coming soon, a self-help guide to complete health!

Made in the USA
Middletown, DE
21 October 2020